DEVELOPMENTAL DISABILITIES:
PSYCHOLOGIC AND SOCIAL IMPLICATIONS

BIRTH DEFECTS: ORIGINAL ARTICLE SERIES
Daniel Bergsma, Series Editor
Volumes in the series published by Alan R. Liss, Inc.

1975

Volume XI, Number 7 — **MORPHOGENESIS AND MALFORMATION OF FACE AND BRAIN**
Jan Langman, *Editor*

1976

Volume XII, Number 1 — **CANCER AND GENETICS**
R. Neil Schimke, Robert L. Summitt, and David J. Harris, *Editors*

Volume XII, Number 3 — **THE EYE AND INBORN ERRORS OF METABOLISM**
Anthony J. Bron and Edward Cotlier, *Editors*

Volume XII, Number 4 — **DEVELOPMENTAL DISABILITIES: PSYCHOLOGIC AND SOCIAL IMPLICATIONS**
Ann E. Pulver, *Editor*

Volume XII, Number 5 — **CYTOGENETICS, ENVIRONMENT AND MALFORMATION SYNDROMES**
R. Neil Schimke, *Editor*

Volume XII, Number 6 — **GROWTH PROBLEMS AND CLINICAL ADVANCES**
R. Neil Schimke, *Editor*

Volume XII, Number 8 — **IRON METABOLISM AND THALASSEMIA**
Anthony Cerami, Charles M. Peterson, and Joseph H. Graziano, *Editors*

IN PRESS

MORPHOGENESIS AND MALFORMATION OF THE LIMB
W. Lenz, *Editor*

THE GENETICS OF HAND MALFORMATIONS
by Victor A. McKusick and Samia Temtamy

MORPHOGENESIS AND MALFORMATION OF THE GENITAL SYSTEM
Richard J. Blandau, *Editor*

The National Foundation – March of Dimes
Birth Defects: Original Article Series, Volume XII, Number 4, 1976

DEVELOPMENTAL DISABILITIES: PSYCHOLOGIC AND SOCIAL IMPLICATIONS

Conference sponsored by
The Johns Hopkins Medical Institutions
School of Hygiene and Public Health
held at
Baltimore, Maryland, March 1–2, 1976

Editors: **Daniel Bergsma, M.D.,** Vice President for Professional Education, The National Foundation
    Ann E. Pulver, M.H.S., The Johns Hopkins University School of Hygiene and Public Health

Associate Editor: **Natalie W. Paul,** The National Foundation
Assistant Editor: **Florence Dickman,** The National Foundation

ALAN R. LISS, INC., NEW YORK, N.Y.

To enhance medical communication in the birth defects field,
The National Foundation publishes the *Birth Defects Atlas and
Compendium*, an *Original Article Series*, *Syndrome Identification*,
a *Reprint Series* and provides a series of films and related brochures.

Further information can be obtained from:

Professional Education Department
The National Foundation — March of Dimes
1275 Mamaroneck Avenue
White Plains, New York 10605

Published by:

Alan R. Liss, Inc.
150 Fifth Avenue
New York, New York 10011

Received for publication July 15, 1976

Copyright © 1976 by The National Foundation

All rights reserved. No part of this publication may be reproduced or transmitted in any form or by any means, electronic or mechanical, including photocopying and recording, or by any information storage and retrieval system, without permission in writing from the copyright holder.

Views expressed in articles published are the authors', and are not to be attributed to The National Foundation or its editors unless expressly so stated.

Library of Congress Cataloging in Publication Data

Main entry under title:

Developmental disabilities — psychologic and social
   implications.

   (Birth defects original article series; v. 12, no. 4)
   Includes bibliographical references.
   1. Handicapped — Congresses. 2. Handicapped —
Psychology — Congresses. I. Bergsma, Daniel. II. Pulver, Ann E.
III. Johns Hopkins University. School of Hygiene and Public Health.
IV. Series. [DNLM: 1. Child development deviations — Congresses.
2. Psychopathology — In infancy and childhood — Congresses.
W1 B1966 v. 12 no. 4 / WS350 D485 1976]
RG626.B63 Vol. 12, no. 4 [HV3000] 616'.043'08s
ISBN 0-8451-1007-1   [362.4]   76-44446

Printed in the United States of America

THE NATIONAL FOUNDATION is dedicated to the long-range goal of preventing birth defects. Our interim goal is to search for ways to ameliorate those birth defects which cannot be prevented.

As a part of our efforts to achieve these goals, we sponsor, or participate in, a variety of scientific meetings and symposia where all questions relating to birth defects are freely discussed. Through our professional education program we speed the dissemination of information by publishing the proceedings of these meetings and symposia. Now and then, in the course of these discussions, individual participants may express personal viewpoints which go beyond the purely scientific in nature and into controversial matters; abortion for example. It should be noted, therefore, that personal viewpoints about such matters will not be censored but obviously this does not constitute an endorsement of them by The National Foundation.

Contents

Contributors ix
Prefatory Note xi
Dedication to Paul V. Lemkau, M.D.
   John C. Hume xii

Introduction
   Ernest M. Gruenberg xv

PART I: MEDICAL ASPECTS

Description of a Handicapped Population:
   The British Columbia Health Surveillance Registry
   James R. Miller 1

PART II: PRE-ADULT DISABILITY: A CHALLENGE TO PSYCHOSOCIAL ADAPTATION

Attitudes and Behavior Toward the Physically Handicapped
   Stephen A. Richardson 15

Research on Families With Handicapped Children — An Aid or an Impediment to Understanding?
   Sheila Hewett 35

The Disabled Child at School: Special Needs and Special Provision
   Elizabeth M. Anderson 47

Adolescence — A Period of Stress, the Search for an Identity
   Thomas E. Strax 63

PART III: INDIVIDUAL AND FAMILY NEEDS

On Deciding the Use of the Family Commons
   Raymond S. Duff 73

Obstacles to Providing Psychologic Services to Disabled Children and Their Families
   Albert J. Solnit 85

Individual and Family Needs in the Health Care of Children with Developmental Disorders
   Ivan B. Pless 91

An Interpretation of the Early Evolution of Care and
  Treatment of Crippled Children in the United States
  Saul Benison 103

PART IV: SOCIETAL REACTION: THE HANDICAPPED INTEGRATED INTO SOCIETY

Education, Recreation, and Vocational Training
  Edmund W. Gordon 119
Alternative Forms of Care for the Disabled:
  Developing Community Services
  Robert Morris. 127
Influence of Litigation on the Lives of the Developmentally
  Disabled: A Preliminary Report
  Kathleen G. Ursin 137
The Making of Public Policy: What Others Do
  With What We Say We Know
  Elizabeth M. Boggs. 149
Adapting Environments for the Developmentally Disabled
  Sandra C. Howell 163
Developmental Disabilities: Educating the Public
  Lowell S. Levin 171
Medical Ecology: The Epidemiology of Handicap
  Leon Eisenberg 181

Contributors

Elizabeth M. Anderson, MA, BSc, PhD [47]
Research Officer
Thomas Coram Research Unit
London WC1N 1A2, England

Saul Benison, PhD [103]
Professor of History and the
   History of Medicine
University of Cincinnati
Cincinnati, OH 45221

Elizabeth M. Boggs, PhD [149]
National Association for
   Retarded Citizens
Washington, DC 20005

Raymond S. Duff, MD, MPH [73]
Department of Pediatrics
Yale University School of Medicine
New Haven, CT 06510

Leon Eisenberg, MD [181]
Professor of Psychiatry
Harvard Medical School and
   Senior Associate in Psychiatry
Children's Hospital Medical Center
Boston, MA 02115

Edmund W. Gordon, EdD [119]
Educational Testing Service
Teachers College, Columbia
   University
New York, NY 10027

Ernest M. Gruenberg, MD, DPH [vx]
Professor and Chairman, Department
   of Mental Hygiene
The Johns Hopkins University
   School of Hygiene and Public Health
Baltimore, MD 21205

Sheila Hewett, PhD [35]
1 Oak Tree Drive
Willow Lane
Gedling, Nottingham, England

Sandra C. Howell, PhD, MPH [163]
Associate Professor, Department
   of Architecture
Massachusetts Institute of
   Technology
Cambridge, MA 02139

Lowell S. Levin, EdD, MPH [171]
Associate Professor, Department of
   Epidemiology and Public Health
Yale University School of Medicine
New Haven, CT 06510

James R. Miller, PhD, FCCMG [1]
Department of Medical Genetics
University of British Columbia
Vancouver, BC V6T 1W5, Canada

Robert Morris, MSC, DSW [127]
Director, Levinson Policy Institute
Kirstein Professor of Social
   Planning
Brandeis University
Waltham, MA 02154

Ivan B. Pless, MD, FRCP (C) [91]
Associate Professor, Department of
   Pediatrics and Epidemiology,
   Health
McGill University and
Director, Community Pediatric
   Research Unit
The Montreal Children's Hospital
Montreal, PQ H3H 1P3, Canada

The number in brackets following each contributor's name is the opening page number of that author's paper.

Stephen A. Richardson, PhD [15]
Professor, Departments of Pediatrics
and Community Health
Albert Einstein College of
Medicine
Bronx, NY 10461

Albert J. Solnit, MD [85]
Sterling Professor of Pediatrics
and Psychiatry
Director, Child Study Center
Yale University
New Haven, CT 06520

Thomas E. Strax, MD [63]
Assistant Medical Director
Moss Rehabilitation Hospital
Assistant Professor of
Rehabilitation Medicine
Temple University School of
Medicine
Philadelphia, PA 19141

Kathleen G. Ursin, MS [137]
Director of Education
The National Center for Law and
the Handicapped, Inc.
South Bend, IN 46617

Prefatory Note

It is our hope that this volume will extend the knowledge and sensitivity of professionals planning for and providing services to persons with developmental disabilities.

Much appreciation and thanks are due to the planning committee for their assistance in arranging this conference: Barton Childs, M.D., Lawrence W. Green, D.P.H., Robert Johnston, M.D., Paul V. Lemkau, M.D., Jonathan P. A. Leopold, M.D., Richard Smith, Ph.D., Leslie Waldman, Virginia Li Wang, Ph.D., and Jerriann Wilson.

We also wish to acknowledge the contributions made by the section chairmen: Dr. Barton Childs, Dr. Julius B. Richmond, Dr. Ronald MacKeith, Dr. Matthew Debuskey, and Alejandro Rodriguez.

Ann E. Pulver, M.H.S.
Conference Director
Doctoral Candidate
Johns Hopkins University
School of Hygiene and Public Health

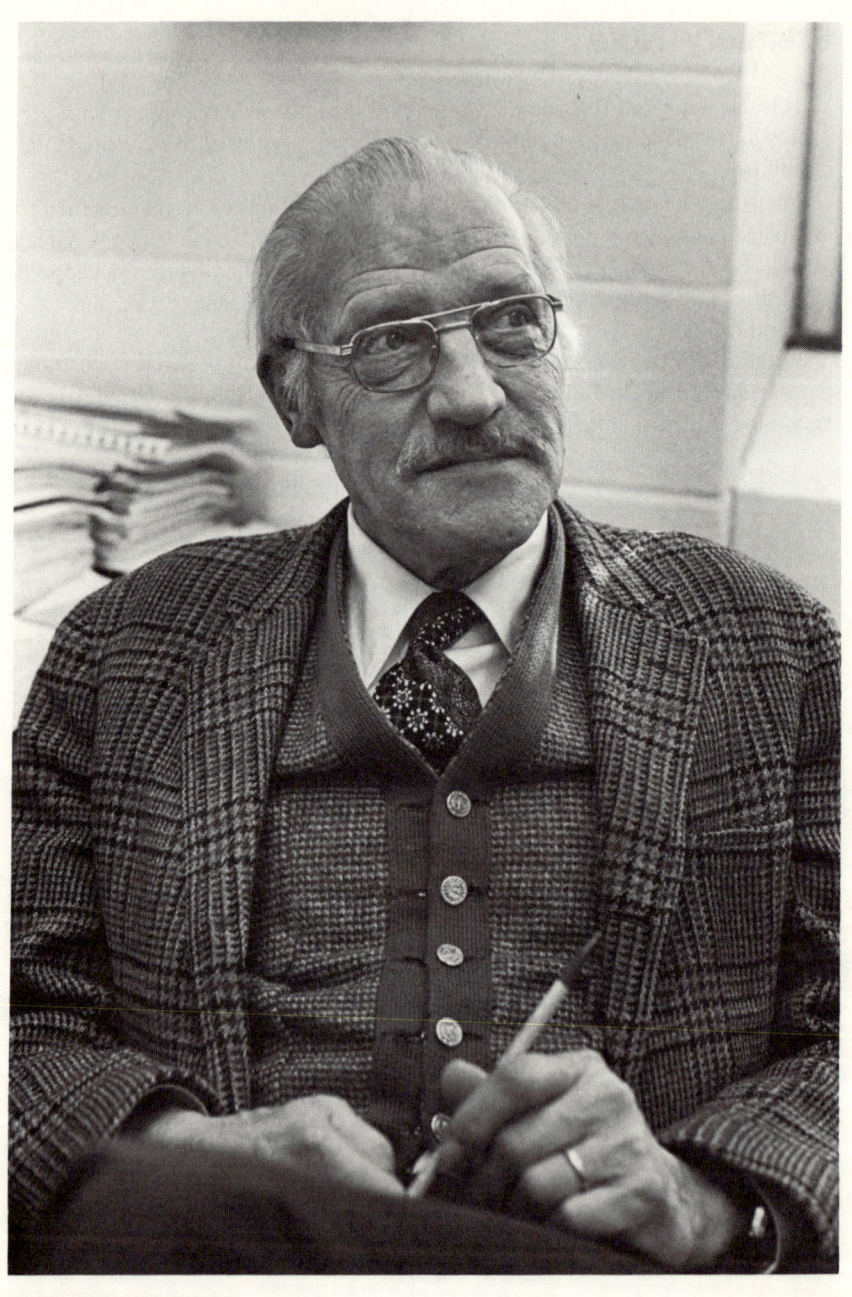

Dedication to Paul V. Lemkau, MD

Over the past 30 years it has been my good fortune to have Dr. Paul Victor Lemkau as my teacher, my colleague and my friend. Thus, it was a particular pleasure for me when the Conference on Developmental Disabilities: Psychologic and Social Implications was convened in his honor.

Dr. Lemkau received his baccalaureate education at Baldwin-Wallace College in Berea, Ohio. His undergraduate medical training was pursued at The Johns Hopkins University School of Medicine. He remained at Hopkins at the Phipps Psychiatric Clinic. While still in his residency training, under the stimulation of and with the encouragement of the great Adolf Meyer, he became interested in the prevention and public health aspects of mental disease. Upon completing his residency training he joined the full-time faculty of The Johns Hopkins School of Hygiene and Public Health. Here he developed the organized program of research and training in mental hygiene which was the first of its kind. It was in this setting and through working with mental and public health agencies that he sharpened the concepts which later were incorporated in the text, "Mental Hygiene in Public Health," which received enthusiastic acclaim and gave great impetus to mental hygiene programs throughout the world.

At the School of Hygiene and Public Health, he headed first a program, then a Division and, since 1961, the Department of Mental Hygiene. He retired from the Chairmanship of the Department at the end of the 1974–75 academic year but remains an active Professor in the Department being involved in the teaching program and in writing up the results of investigations which have been underway for the past several years.

All who are familiar with the field of mental hygiene know of the many leadership roles he has played: as head of the Mental Hygiene Division of the Maryland State Department of Health and later as the first Commissioner of Mental Health in New York City; as a stimulator and leader of the voluntary mental health movement; as advisor to every level of government including both civilian and military agencies; and as a pioneering investigator and teacher. It is little wonder that he has been referred to as the "Father of Mental Hygiene."

Those who have had the privilege of being faculty colleagues or students of his are well aware of contributions such as those listed above. However, he is best known to them for his ready accessibility to individuals and ideas, his breadth of interest, his wise counseling, his high standards of performance in both professional and personal matters, or in sum and most importantly, as a thoroughly fine and decent human.

In view of his devotion to the fields of mental hygiene and public health and his recognition of the implications for these of the subject matter incorporated in this volume, it is fitting that this work be dedicated to him. The excellent, penetrating papers presented by the distinguished roster of authors represent a worthy tribute to a meritorious teacher, physician, and scientist.

John C. Hume, MD, DPH
Dean, Johns Hopkins University
School of Hygiene and Public Health

Introduction

Ernest M. Gruenberg, MD, DPH

Developmental disabilities emerge from handicaps following a faulty development of the individual organism. The person experiences a disability for any given level of handicap which is determined by the way that handicapped person interacts with the society of which he is a part. We have learned a great deal in the last 30 years, I believe, about how to reduce the functional disability without yet knowing how in many situations to correct the handicap or defect in the organism.

So our fight against these disabilities, developmental disabilities, has two sides to it. On the one hand we gradually, very slowly, succeed in finding preventable causes for them. For example, very few severely rickettsial children are seen today. Such progress is made through research and organized public health efforts to interrupt the processes by which infections or injuries or poisons or a deficiency of nutrition or nurture or a defect of gene makeup produces the handicaps we worry about. When the multiple paths to the many handicaps look terribly complicated, it is very helpful to realize that all the discoveries about preventable causes of these conditions fall into five categories: infections, injuries, poisons, nutritional deficiency or defective genes. Developmental defects result from these kinds of causes operating during the individual's development at sometime between conception and maturity.

When we fail to prevent a defect, however, we must ask what we can do so that the individual may live a life with a minimum of disability. The two institutions of Johns Hopkins — the great hospital and a great school of public health — complement each other. The bigger, the more voluminous, the more energetic in day to day obvious activities is the hospital which responds to the failures of public health to prevent disease. Public health will continue to fail.

xvi / Introduction

It's a never-ending fight. We'll always have disease and while prevention is better than cure, there will always be people who need cure; and there will always be patients who need special services to make the best out of the preventive failures. Because medical research has made certain types of progress, this field of work paradoxically is becoming more and more important. While we have made little progress in preventing developmental defects, technical advances in treatment have developed cures for the fatal complications of developmental defects which led to death early in infancy and childhood a few decades ago. As a result, the proportion of the total population which has developed mental defects is growing constantly. The life span of people with defects is getting longer and longer.

The volume of work that society must do to identify the nature of the handicap and define the disability in the narrowest possible terms grows. We also must diagnose the social problems — society's problems — in helping each individual who comes into society to occupy a satisfying role.

I
MEDICAL ASPECTS

1
MEDICAL ASPECTS

Description of a Handicapped Population: The British Columbia Health Surveillance Registry

James R. Miller, PhD, FCCMG

In discussing the size and range of problems of mental health we approach the issue of how they are spread in the population and how many of them we must be prepared, in some way or another, to take care of. — Dr. Paul V. Lemkau [1].

Dr. Lemkau's statement is taken from the first page of the first of 6 lectures with the overall title, *Basic Issues in Psychiatry*, published in 1959. The first chapter is concerned with "the size and range of mental health problems." It is refreshing to see first things placed first and not relegated to the last chapter or as an afterthought in an appendix. Although it may seem patently obvious that definition of the size and extent of a health problem should precede an attempt to resolve it, it is surprising how frequently this aspect is ignored while everyone scurries about resolving undefined problems.

It often surprises both my biology and medical students, who have been brought up in modern biology, to realize that we still do not know how to count human beings with specific disabilities in order to obtain reliable incidence or prevalence rates. It always astounds them that we may know a great deal about the genetics, biochemistry, and biophysics of a disease and yet have no sound idea of how many individuals have this disease, what their problems are, and how we should adequately provide for their needs. We have ample means of recording mortality, because death is legally a reportable event and death records contain information on cause of death. However, no such legal requirements exist for obtaining morbidity statistics. From time to time different societies believe that a disease (or a group of diseases) is sufficiently important to require legal reporting, eg infectious diseases and cancer. It is also possible to get hospitalization statistics, but these are highly biased and often give an irrelevant picture of the true needs of a population of handicapped. Special surveys can be conducted, but they too have limited value. They are often expensive to initiate, and their value lasts for a relatively short period of time.

I would like to return to Dr. Lemkau's lecture for a moment. In it, he is concerned not only with the magnitude, but also with the diversity of psychiatric disabilities, each with characteristic epidemiologic features, requirements for services, and so on. He stresses the importance of recognizing the plural terms "illnesses" and "diseases" rather than the singular, which masks the specificity of separate types of disease. In this particular conference, our concern is with handicapping illnesses, and we must recognize that they cannot be grouped and that each type must be considered separately because of specific and, very often, individualistic needs.

In this presentation, I should like to extend some of these ideas of Dr. Lemkau and describe one system that is attempting to define a population of handicapped individuals.

THE B.C. HEALTH SURVEILLANCE REGISTRY

History

The history and basic operational procedures of the B.C. Registry have been described in detail [2], and Table I summarizes some of the key points. The changes in name reflect definite policy changes. The 1950 survey indicated that there were many handicapped children with unmet needs, hence, the first definition of the criteria for registration was "any child under 21 years of age who has a disability severe enough to interfere with normal living, obtaining an education and later earning a livelihood." However, as many of the individuals on the register reached the age of 21 and were still disabled, it seemed foolish to simply drop them. Hence, in 1962, the change of name was made and the criteria were enlarged to include "a person who possesses a long term physical, mental and/or emotional problem which is likely to be permanently disabling, interfere with his/her education or prevent full and open employment." In 1962 these criteria were modified to include "any person with a familial condition or congenital malformation which is not disabling." Finally, in 1974, this Handicap Register was merged administratively with a cancer register and several risk

TABLE 1. History of B. C. Registry

1948 — Federal health grants made available to provinces
1950 — Survey in B. C. reveals many handicapped children with unmet needs
1952 — Crippled Children's Registry established
1960 — Registry for Handicapped Children and Adults
1975 — B. C. Health Surveillance Registry

registers under the heading B.C. Health Surveillance Registry. Since the Handicap Register reflects its historic beginnings, the bulk of the cases are still children or adults who were registered as children. The staff of the registry recognizes this deficiency and tries constantly to correct it. Three examples that have occurred during the past year will illustrate how the basic registry structure can be adapted to meet specific needs. First, the Provincial Department of Human Resources, which is responsible for payments of support to handicapped adults, asked the registry to enroll its total caseload in order to obtain a better idea of the location and nature of special rehabilitative facilities which might be required in the province. This is being carried out at present and will increase the number of adult cases on the register. Second, the registry has been asked to play a central role in coordinating the services of spinal cord injuries in the province. Finally, the registry has been asked to serve as the base for a "stroke" register. (This has not been implemented at present.) To those of us who have been associated with the registry for many years, these are encouraging signs that more individuals and organizations are recognizing the value of proper enumeration, follow-up, and coordination of services to handicapped adults.

Throughout the evolutionary changes outlined in Table 1, the registry has been administered by the Division of Vital Statistics of the Health Department of the Province. While it never has been stated as such, implicit in this administrative structure is the clear indication that health statistics are, or should be, part of the routine documentation of a society. This administrative base has other important consequences which I shall mention later.

The Province of B.C. had a population of approximately 1.5 million when the registry was formed and now has 2.5 million. Although the area is approximately 360,000 sq miles, much of it is mountainous, and close to half the population resides in the southwest corner near the border of the United States.

Ascertainment of Cases

From the beginning, the registry has used multiple sources of ascertainment and while initially case finding was limited to individuals under 21 years for the past 12 years it has not been restricted to any specific age group. The sources of ascertainment are outlined in Table 2. No registry system can guarantee total enumeration, but we believe multiple ascertainment is the best method to use, and it provides good estimates of true incidence and prevalence rates. As of December 31, 1975 there were over 75,000 cases on the register.*

Operations

The daily operations of data processing of the registry are outlined elsewhere and are not essential to this presentation, except to state that the ICDA codes

---

*These data do not include cancer cases which are kept on a separate register and are not being used in this presentation.

TABLE 2. Sources of Ascertainment in B. C. Registry

A. From beginning:
1. Physician's Notice of Birth — must be completed within 48 hr of birth. Useful source of data on major surface defects present at birth.
2. Public Health Units — generalized public health program including schools and special institutions for the handicapped.
3. Special Treatment Centers — pediatric out-patient and diagnostic clinics, genetic counseling units, specialty clinics for mental retardation, rehabilitation units, etc.
4. Voluntary Health Agencies — such as Canadian Arthritis Society, Canadian National Institute for the Blind.
5. Private Physicians — useful in rare instances, but not a good source in general.

B. Since 1964:
6. Stillbirth Registration — valuable data for incidence rates on major congenital defects.
7. Death Registration (of children under 6 years) — provides data for incidence rates on many conditions of childhood.
8. Obstetrical Discharge Summary — a form completed on all deliveries in 3 major obstetric units in Vancouver; provides data for incidence rates on malformations detected within first 5 days of life.
9. Discharge diagnoses of all hospital admissions (of those born in 1964 and later) — potentially of great value for all classes of handicapping disabilities. (Not put into operation until 1966).

C. 1975 and future:
10. Department of Human Resources — all disabled individuals who receive benefits from the province.
11. Specialty Clinics for Disabled Adults — eg stroke, spinal cord injuries.

are used with some special modifications in certain categories. The coding forms on each individual have provision for 4 disabilities. These are coded separately or as a syndrome (if the anomalies are consistent with one). In reports on the registry, data are presented by number of disabilities or groups of disabilities and/or by number of affected individuals. In addition, an etiology code has been developed and is used for each case.

Uses of Registry Data

The data on the register have been used in many ways, but I will confine my remarks to 3 examples which keep to my task of defining a handicapped population: 1) the profile of a disability load in the child and adult populations; 2) some incidence and prevalence data; 3) follow-up studies.

The profile of a disability load in children and adults. Table 3 presents a comparison of the 10 most frequent disabilities amongst children alone and amongst children and adult cases on the register at the end of 1974. The profile of the children's disabilities is probably quite an accurate reflection of problems in the community. However, the adult load, while valuable, obviously has some

TABLE 3. Ten of the Most Frequent Disabilities of Children and Adults, and of Children Only (Under 20) Among Live Cases on Register at Year-end, 1974 (Excluding persons known to be resident outside of B.C.)

Children and adults			Children only		
Disability category (in descending order) with ICDA code number	No. of persons	% total (57,841)	Disability category (in descending order) with ICDA code number	No. of children	% total (31,707)
Mental retardation (310–315)	3,763	15.2	Strabismus (373)	4,964	15.7
Strabismus (373)	6,590	11.4	Mental retardation (310–315)	3,982[a]	12.6
Rheumatoid arthritis (712.0–712.3)	4,340[b]	7.5	Congenital anomalies of heart and circulatory system (746, 747)	2,962	9.3
Congenital anomalies of heart and circulatory system (746, 747)	3,931	6.8	Clubfoot (754)	2,434	7.7
Epilepsy (345)	3,627	6.3	Epilepsy (345)	1,985	6.3
Blindness (379)	3,083	5.3	Cerebral paralysis (343, 344)	1,489[c]	4.7
Cerebral paralysis (343, 344)	3,000	5.2	Congenital dislocation of hip (755.6)	1,413	4.5
Clubfoot (754)	2,810	4.9			
Impaired hearing and deafness (389)	2,603	4.5	Impaired hearing and deafness (389)	1,343	4.2
Speech disturbance (781.5)	2,343	4.2	Cleft lip and/or palate (749)	1,268	4.0
			Speech disturbance (781.5)	1,178	3.7

[a]Includes 779 children with Down syndrome
[b]Includes 267 children
[c]Includes 1,268 children with cerebral spastic infantile paralysis (code 343)

serious gaps, eg stroke sequelae and mental illness. The data on strokes might be forthcoming, but the data on mental illness present a problem to which I will return.

Incidence and prevalence data. Over the years, the registry has provided information for the determination of incidence and prevalence rates for a variety of handicapping illnesses. While absolute numbers are important in planning, the incidence and prevalence rates are useful in providing a basis for planning on the returns of such programs as screening. Also, if broken down into such things as age-specific rates, it can give a good idea of changes that will affect planning. I should like to give, as an example, a recent study by my colleague, Dr. Brian Lowry and his associates, on Down syndrome [3]. In this study, cases of Down syndrome on the register were linked with birth registration forms in order to obtain maternal age. Mean maternal age declined for both normal children and Down syndrome children during the period studied, 1952–1973. During this period the mean maternal age for all live births declined from 27.4 to 25.9 years, and the mean maternal age for Down syndrome decreased from 34.1 to 28.1 years. As a consequence, 80% of Down syndrome children were born to women under 35 in 1972–73, whereas 20 years ago 46% of cases were born to women in this age group. It was this latter figure that gave rise to the statement that the number of cases of Down syndrome could be cut in half if women over 35 did not reproduce and, of course, amniocentesis programs began with such a goal, implicitly or explicitly stated. Obviously, the ground rules have changed. Only 20% of cases now occur in this maternal age group, and in order to detect 50% of cases, a maternal age cut-off under 30 would have to be instituted. Obviously, this would have profound consequences on the distribution of health resources. I am not going to comment on this but refer anyone interested to a recent report on this topic [4]. Of course, this example is not exactly applicable to our problem, because the implications are for the procedure of amniocentesis and not for planning for long-term support for handicapped populations, but I believe they demonstrate my point — namely, that it is important to be aware of changes that are occurring in populations if intelligent planning is to be executed.

Follow-up. Many registers have foundered on the issue of follow-up. Although such registers can define methods of ascertainment and have reliable intake diagnosis, there is no mechanism for follow-up. Hence, the register in time becomes full of files on individuals whose whereabouts and current health status are unknown. Because of this, many public health administrators have shunned all types of registers as well intentioned and theoretically sound but in practice of little value because of the real threat of stagnation.

Description of a Handicapped Population / 7

From the outset, the administrators of the B.C. Registry have been aware of this hazard and have actively pursued follow-up procedures. The use of multiple sources of ascertainment without age restriction assures some degree of follow-up, because information on second and third registrations of an individual permit monitoring and evaluation of diagnosis, the addition of new diagnoses, changes in diagnoses, and the possibility of following the natural history of certain diseases. In some cases on which further information is desired, routine follow-up is instituted by registry personnel. In order to ensure a more comprehensive follow-up of cases, a systematic follow-up of all individuals who became 7 or 14 years of age in a given year was initiated several years ago. These 2 ages were chosen because 7-year-olds have been in school for 2 years and, hence, learning disabilities would probably have become manifest, while the 14-year-old group is only a year away from legal school-leaving age. The public health units throughout the province were used to collect the data. Each unit was sent forms and asked to report on those patients known to it. The form was a shocking pink to attract attention and was made simple in order to maximize returns.

The results of the first 5 years of this follow-up have been published [5]. I am not going to detail results but simply point out some of the high spots, using 1973 data as an example. The data in Table 4 demonstrate the amazing effort of the public health personnel in this follow-up. The 97.5% of forms returned and the 81% completion is in good agreement with other years. The failure to obtain completed forms on all cases is disappointing but not surprising in a mobile population. Some of these lost cases are individuals who have moved out of the province, while others are individuals in the large metropolitan area of Vancouver where follow-up is more difficult. The impressive part of the follow-up is the consistency from year to year and between the 2 age groups. Since 1967, the percentage of cases with residual handicap in both age groups has been around 66. As might be expected, this varies greatly with the type of disability, being close to 100% for mental retardation and quite low for those categories of congenital defects which are correctable by surgery. The data in Table 5 illustrate another consistent observation, namely, the type of schooling required by the 2 age groups. In both instances, 75% of the cases are in the regular school system. Of those not in regular school, 11% in both categories are in schools for the retarded. In the group of 7-year-olds, 10% are in special classes and 3% are in "other schools." In the 14-year-old groups, the percentage in special classes drops to 5% and the percentage in other schools increases to 7%. This change reflects a movement in the older age group from formal special classes into classes oriented toward such programs as workshops and special opportunity classes. Information that has been interesting but, unfortunately, not used effectively,

TABLE 4. Summary of Returns From the Age 7 and 14 Follow-up Survey, 1973

	Number	%
Forms returned	2,020	97.5
Forms completed	1,670	81.1
Total in survey	2,071	100

TABLE 5. Schooling of 7- and 14-Year-Olds With Residual Handicap

	7-year-olds		14-year-olds	
	No.	%	No.	%
Regular school class	529	75	737	75
Special class	71	10	52	5
School for retarded	77	11	103	11
Other schools	17	3	68	7
Not attending school	8	1	18	2
Total	702	100	978	100

relates to the number of 14-year-olds who will need some special job placement when they complete schooling. In each group this has been over 50% of those with residual handicaps.

The lesson seems clear: The consistency from year to year and from age group to age group means that long-term planning for the minimal needs of the handicapped can be based on the population of 7-year-olds. No attempt has been made to initiate this type of follow-up for older groups because of the difficulties until now of handling the adult population. However, these difficulties may soon be at an end and similar follow-ups on older groups may be possible.

Future

Recently, someone whose opinion I value, stated that the B.C. Registry was unique and that it was not exportable because of this unique history and the personalities involved with its establishment for over 20 years. I found this opinion sobering but cannot accept it. Any success the registry has achieved is based on the fact that it has been kept flexible. The data presented in Tables 1 and 2 demonstrate this. New techniques and programs have been developed over the years, and new proposals for the use of the data are constantly evaluated. Every effort is made to avoid stagnation. Therefore, it is appropriate to ask about the future. How can the registry develop? It is possible to speculate at length on this topic but I will confine my comments to two areas — namely, improvement in the registration of adults, and record linkage.

Adults. Although historically the registry has focused on children's diseases, this focus has gradually broadened to include adult disabilities. It is obvious that there are serious gaps in the registration of adults (Table 3). The increased interest in the use of the registry by those individuals and organizations concerned with disabled adults bodes well, but this aspect of the registry program will require a great deal of effort.

Record linkage. Since the registry is part of the Division of Vital Statistics it is possible to link files within it to other vital records such as births, marriages, and death. At present, this can be done manually, but machine methods for such linkage have been developed by Howard Newcombe and his colleagues at Atomic Energy of Canada Limited at Chalk River, Ontario [6, 7]. These techniques have not been implemented routinely but are being considered, and the registry is in the process of arranging for the appointment of Dr. Benjamin Trimble as a record linkage consultant. One of the first steps in any linkage project of the registry would involve linking the files on the handicapped register, which have been the concern of this presentation, with the files of the cancer register. For reasons which cannot be enumerated here, the cancer register has superb diagnostic information but identification data are poor in terms of linkability.

To have all registry files as part of a large linkage network will be a great benefit and will increase its service and research potential immeasurably.

Problems

There are many problems associated with the day-to-day management of such a registry system. In general, these problems involve the methods by which reliable information flows continuously into the system and important, useful data flow out to those whose cooperation is essential to the success of the system.

In addition to these difficulties, I want to discuss 2 problems which I believe are of major importance, namely, the failure to obtain adequate registration on mental illnesses and the constant need to protect confidentiality of the records.

Failure to obtain registration on mental illness are complicated, but the chief reasons are outlined by Dr. Lemkau in the lecture to which I referred earlier. He states, "The fact that we deal in symptoms so frequently, and symptoms which may represent many kinds of etiology, does detract somewhat from the idea of specificity in psychiatric diseases." An additional problem, which Dr. Lemkau perhaps implies but does not discuss, is that there is great concern on the part of those in the mental health field with the fact that the registry puts labels on people. As I have repeatedly pointed out, the registry does not label. The label is put on by those who register.

Frankly, after grappling with this problem of mental illness for over a decade, I do not see an obvious solution short of thought revolution on the part of those in the mental health field. Somehow, they must see that the proper understanding of a health problem begins with a definition that must include a statement of the magnitude and nature of the disease. And while classifications tend to convey a sense of definition that may not exist in reality, some type of categorization is necessary for adequate enumeration.

In many instances, the problem of registering mental illness is based on concern for the confidentiality of the records in the register. The need to maintain the security of records is a constant requirement of anyone who maintains large data systems. There are 3 factors in the B.C. Registry that guarantee the confidentiality of the files. First, since the registry is part of the Division of Vital Statistics, all persons are trained to respect the information which they handle daily. Graduate students and others who use the records for special projects are sworn to an oath of secrecy. In themselves, these procedures are no guarantee of confidentiality, but they do impress upon those who use the records the importance of maintaining the security. Second, there is an amendment to the Provincial Evidence Act which protects those who register, those who are registered, and those who use the data on the registry. In addition, all of the information on the registry is "declared to be privileged communications which may not be used, offered, or received in evidence in any legal proceeding at any time." (The entire section of the act is published in Ref. 2.) Finally, the registry personnel never has direct contact with any registered person. Follow-up for any reason is carried out through the person or agency who registers the case. If direct contact is required, then permission for this is obtained through the registering agency. Statistics are provided to anyone who makes a legitimate request, but requests involving names of individuals, whether contact is desired or not, are handled in a very rigorous way involving screening by a committee.

CONCLUSIONS

The problems with which this conference is concerned are formidable, and their resolution is not going to come from any one source. My contribution has developed from the thesis that the first step on the path is a proper understanding of the number and nature of the affected individuals. The B.C. Registry appears to be a useful tool for this purpose, but I close with some cautionary observations. After 20 years of operation, the registry is still not completely successful;

there are many gross deficiencies in ascertainment, some of which I have enumerated, and the data on the registry are not used effectively by those who should use them for proper health planning. I believe that each health area, whether it be province, state, city, or country, must develop its own methods for evaluating the number and needs of the handicapped individual within its jurisdiction. Perhaps my colleague, whose comment I mentioned earlier, is correct and the formal registry structure in B.C. is not exportable, but I do hope that those of you who are concerned with these issues can benefit to some extent from our experience.

REFERENCES

1. Lemkau, P. V.: "Basic Issues in Psychiatry." Springfield: Charles C Thomas, 1959.
2. Lowry, R. B., Miller, J. R., Scott, A. E., and Renwick, D. H. G.: The British Columbia Registry for Handicapped Children and Adults: Evolutionary changes over twenty years. Can. J. Public Health 66:322, 1975.
3. Lowry, R. B., Jones, D. C., Renwick, D. H. G., and Trimble, B. K.: Down syndrome in British Columbia 1952–1973: Incidence and mean maternal age. (Accepted for publication, Teratology, 1975.)
4. Stein, Z., Susser, M., and Guterman, A. V.: Screening program for prevention of Down syndrome. Lancet 1:305, 1973.
5. Miller, J. R., and Gallagher, R. P.: The use of a Registry caseload survey in establishing rehabilitative needs of the handicapped. J. Ment. Defic. Res. 19:101, 1975.
6. Newcombe, H. B.: Present state and long-term objectives of the British Columbia population study. In "Proceedings of the 3rd International Congress of Human Genetics." Baltimore: The Johns Hopkins Press, 1967.
7. Smith, M. E., and Newcombe, H. B.: Methods for computer linkage of hospital admission-separation records into cumulative health histories. Methods Inf. Med. 14:118, 1975.

II
PRE-ADULT DISABILITY:
A CHALLENGE TO PSYCHOSOCIAL ADAPTATION

Attitudes and Behavior Toward the Physically Handicapped

Stephen A. Richardson, PhD

Now that there have been about 30 years of research dealing with the social consequences of physical disability it is time to do some stocktaking. What have been the main directions of research? What methods have been used? To what extent are findings consistent or contradictory? How good is the evidence on which findings are based? How can findings be made useful? I shall try to look at some of these questions, but within the compass of a paper the presentation must necessarily be selective and reflect a personal view. The focus will be primarily on research related to the attitude and behavior of persons who are not disabled toward those who are.

PERSONALITY AND ATTITUDE RESEARCH

The early research related to physical disability is well summed up by the title of an early review, *Adjustment to Physical Handicap and Illness: A Survey of the Social Psychology of Physique and Disability (1953)* [1]. The studies were psychologic in conception, focused on the handicapped person, and reflected a strong personality orientation. For example, there was interest in whether particular personality types were associated with particular kinds of physical handicaps. In general, this approach did not prove productive.

Somewhat later in the 1950s–1960s, psychologists studied attitudes toward the disabled. H. E. Yuker and his associates in 1966 developed an "Attitudes Toward Disabled Persons" scale [2], which was subsequently borrowed by other investigators.

Subjects were asked to react to a series of statements such as, "Disabled persons are usually friendly," or "Disabled people are often less aggressive than normal people." No information was given to the subjects about the kind of disability or the kind of person who was disabled in terms of age, sex, or any other characteristic. The term "disabled" was not defined, and no attempt was made to determine what the term conjured up for each subject. Some of the results using this scale were: 1) females have more positive attitudes toward the disabled than males; 2) with increasing grade-school education, attitudes become less favorable, but then become more favorable with additional schooling; 3) positive attitudes are related to acceptance of persons who are "different"; and 4) increased equal-status contact is related to more positive attitudes.

Siller and his associates [3] became dissatisfied with the term "disabled" and added a measure of specificity by obtaining attitudes toward blindness, amputation, and cosmetic handicaps. Examples of their findings are that ego strength and security are positively associated with acceptance of the handicapped, while anxiety, hostility, and rigidity were negatively correlated. The variability in response of subjects to handicapped persons is an important theoretic and practical issue that has largely been ignored in research which focuses on interpersonal behavior between persons with and without handicaps.

VALUE RESEARCH

Richardson and his colleagues [4–12] used pictures of handicapped children to learn about reactions to a variety of physical handicaps. All the characteristics of the children in the pictures were held constant except the presence or absence of a visible physical handicap and the kind of handicap. The pictures used are shown in Figure 1. Subjects were shown same-sex pictures. They were asked to look carefully at the pictures which were laid out before them in a random order. After they had done this they were asked, "Which boy (or girl) do you like best?" When the subject indicated the response, generally by pointing, the picture chosen was removed, and the subject was then asked, "Now, which boy (or girl) do you like best?" After the subject indicated his or her choice that picture was then removed, and the procedure was repeated until only one picture remained. The procedure obtained the subject's order of preference. Expression of preference is essentially the expression of values. The following examples of results indicate the kinds of questions which were explored:

1) With subjects ranging in age from 6 to adult, a large majority of all groups liked the picture of the child without a visible handicap best.

2) There was remarkable degree of agreement as to which handicaps are more and less preferred. At ages 8–10 the order from the most to least liked was: leg brace and crutches, children in wheel chair, amputation of the forearm, facial disfigurement, obesity.

3) Children who were physically handicapped agreed in their preference orders with children who were not.

Attitudes Toward the Handicapped / 17

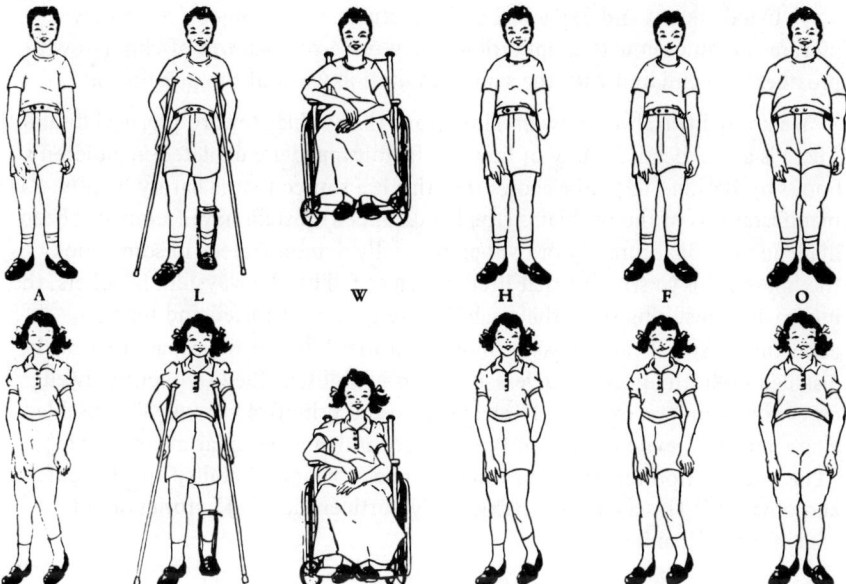

Fig. 1.

4) In general boys showed less preference for handicaps that interfered with physical activities than did girls; whereas girls showed less preference for handicaps which were cosmetic and interfered with social relations than did boys.

5) There was more conformity to the average preference order among girls than boys.

6) A general preference ordering became apparent by age 6.

7) Changes occurred in preference for different handicaps between the ages of 5 and adulthood. a) The child with a leg brace and crutches and the child in the wheelchair were more liked by subjects with increasing age. b) The child with a forearm amputation and the child with a facial disfigurement became less liked, but the change occurred more markedly around the onset of puberty. c) As children grew older their preference rank order became increasingly close to the parent of the same sex.

8) To determine the relative salience of skin color and physical disability, these 2 variables were systematically varied in the pictures. It was found that physical handicap was so powerful a cue that it largely masked preferences based on skin color.

9) In a different and expanded set of pictures, when subjects were shown pictures of children with amputations, they preferred pictures of children with prostheses to children with the same amputation without the prosthesis.

We know little about how children learn their values toward physical disability. There is a provocative study of how the handicapped are depicted in children's books by Baskin [13]. She shows that this is a source that is hardly helpful. "The manifestations of the problems (the handicapped) sustain have frequently been inadequately, inaccurately or over-emotionally demonstrated. In some books the 'message' is so strident that literary values fall by the wayside. In others, the incapacities resulting from the disability are grossly distorted and tend to caricature." Specifically, Baskin finds the stories "distort the capabilities of the disabled by both under and overestimation of abilities, they frequently dwell on cruelties and are excessively melancholy and primitive in tone. The disabled character's home life is frequently portrayed as being irregular in structure." "The interrelationship between violence, rejection and disability are clearcut and obvious." This analysis is particularly pertinent in 25/45 stories about some form of handicap.

RESEARCH ON INITIAL REACTIONS TO THE HANDICAPPED

Babies' Responses to a 3-Dimensional Model of a Human Face

We have thus far looked at studies where the stimuli used were words and pictures. Kagan et al [14] elicited responses of 4-month-old babies to somewhat more complex stimuli. In one condition the infants were shown a 3-dimensional human face with the features in normal position. In the second condition the infants were shown the same face but the position of the features were changed, eg the nose was placed where an eye should have been. Infants who saw the face with abnormal placement of the features responded with anxiety, fear, and crying. The study suggests that very early in life we develop a set of expectations of what is characteristic of a human face.

Initial Social Encounter Between a Handicapped and Nonhandicapped Person

There have been a number of experimental studies of interpersonal relations between handicapped and nonhandicapped persons. They have dealt with the question of whether persons who are not handicapped alter their behavior in the presence of someone who has a visible handicap. To hold constant all factors except handicap, the studies use a confederate of the experimenter who was not handicapped, but who, in some instances, appeared handicapped. In one series of studies this was done by simulating a leg amputation through the use of a wheel chair with a false bottom, where the leg was covered below the knee. The studies deal with a short interaction between 2 persons who have never met. Using this design Kleck et al [15] found that subjects who interacted with the person appearing handicapped 1) exhibited more anxiety, 2) distorted their opinions in ways they felt would be more acceptable to the handicapped person, 3) were less spontaneous, 4) showed less variability in the opinions they offered, and 5) terminated the meeting sooner. In a later study, Kleck [16] also found the nonhandicapped subjects generally inhibited their gestures. The results support the concept of Kelley et al [17] who suggested that in an initial social encounter with persons with a handicap, there is a feeling of ambivalence, resulting in behavior that is inhibited and formal in order to conceal negative feelings which may cause embarrassment.

The question of ambivalence toward those who are handicapped was examined by Katz et al [18]. In an experimental study, they showed that under conditions where subjects had ambivalent feelings and behaved unpleasantly toward a confederate of the experimenter who appeared as physically handicapped, subjects later denigrated the handicapped person in order to deal with the guilt they felt about their negative behavior.

The Reaction of Mothers to the Birth of a Handicapped Child

In a study by Strasser and Sievert [19] of babies born with limb deformities, the mothers reported violent reactions of grief, depression, social withdrawal, and an initial preoccupation with the limb deformity, in some cases to such a degree that they were unable to respond to the other characteristics and behavior of their baby. Drotar et al [20] found that following the birth of a handicapped child, parents reported feelings of shock, denial, sadness, and anger followed by a period of adaptation and reorganization. Hunt [21], in a series of interviews with mothers of children with myelomeningocele, found that "mothers described the overwhelming shock when first told of the baby's defect, their isolation from the baby they had waited to see and hold and from husband and relations who . . . were sometimes afraid to meet the mother." Roskies [22] in a study in Canada of mothers of children born with limb deformities, found that both parents and professionals were at a loss as to how to behave, and all the usual ritual activities following the birth of the child were completely disrupted. The severity of the crisis was evident 3 to 4 years later when most of the mothers, in recalling the birth, broke down and sobbed.

Experiences in Initial Social Encounters Reported by Persons With Physical Handicaps

Davis [23] interviewed informants who were visibly handicapped. He points out, "even if only superficially, one is expected to remain oriented to the whole person and to avoid the expression of a precipitous or fixed concern with any single attribute of his, however noteworthy or laudable it may be. . . . The handicapped person in many cases cannot control his appearance sufficiently so that its striking particularity will not call a certain amount of attention to itself."

Whether or not the handicap is responded to overtly "the underlying condition of heightened, narrowed awareness causes the interaction to be articulated too excessively in terms of it." "Handicapped informants report familiar signs of discomfort and stickiness: the guarded references, the common everyday words suddenly made taboo, the fixed stare elsewhere, the artificial levity, the compulsive loquaciousness, the awkward solemnity." Davis also points out that the initial rules of social interaction enable the handicapped person to be accorded a fictional acceptance, the surface acceptance democratic manners guarantee to nearly all.

In autobiographies by people who are disabled there are accounts of difficulties, embarrassments, and humiliation experienced in initial social encounters [24–26].

All the different types of studies that have been reviewed so far deal with initial reactions to physical disability, reactions to attitude scales, to pictures, to 3-dimensional representations of handicaps, and reactions in initial social encounters. The results from this wide range of studies suggest some tentative generalizations. The first set of generalizations deals with the reactions of those who are not handicapped:

1) Initial reactions toward those who are physically handicapped are less favorable than toward those who are not handicapped.

2) There is considerable agreement among subcultures as to which physical handicaps are more or less preferred.

3) Emotional arousal and anxiety occur in varying degrees in an initial encounter with a handicapped person.

4) Reactions described in 1–3 above are present early in childhood.

5) The physical disability initially dominates the attention of the nonhandicapped person. The salience of the handicap leads to inattention to the other attributes of the handicapped person — attributes which normally would be included in initial interpersonal evaluation and used in guiding the initial stages of the interpersonal relationship.

6) The initial interaction frequently includes a feeling of ambivalence on the part of the nonhandicapped person. For fear of revealing the negative aspect of the ambivalence, the nonhandicapped person is more formal and controlled in the behavior he or she exhibits.

7) Depending on the experience in the initial social encounter, the ambivalence felt may later be expressed as denigration of the handicapped or as giving overly favorable impressions.

8) There is inhibition of nonverbal behavior, such as gesture, and a tendency to come less close physically.

9) The nonhandicapped exhibit less variability in their behavior, and they dis-

tort their opinions in the directions they feel are more acceptable to the handicapped person.

10) The nonhandicapped tend to terminate the initial social encounter more quickly with a handicapped than with a nonhandicapped person.

11) The reaction of a parent to the birth of a child with a visible handicap includes some of the characteristics already described, but in addition includes shock, denial, grieving, social withdrawal, and depression.

The second set of tentative generalizations deal with the consequences of the reactions described for those who are physically handicapped:

1) In a social gathering where individuals have not previously met, the handicapped person is likely to be the recipient of fewer social contacts. Negative and ambivalent feelings in the nonhandicapped may lead them to avoid social encounters with the handicapped, especially when there are other nonhandicapped people in the group from which to choose and when the nonhandicapped have greater mobility than the handicapped.

2) The handicapped person is at a disadvantage if his impairment initially becomes a focus of attention. It is difficult for him to present other attributes of himself which may gain attention and form the basis for developing a social relationship.

3) The combination of anxiety, ambivalence, and formalization of behavior in the nonhandicapped person result in the handicapped person not experiencing as wide a range of behavior as the nonhandicapped. In the case of babies born with a handicap, the early mother-child relationship may be severely disrupted.

4) The distortion of information given the handicapped person by the nonhandicapped person, because he does not wish to offend or hurt the handicapped person, will result in the handicapped person not obtaining honest feedback when he behaves inappropriately. This reduces the likelihood of learning the appropriateness and inappropriateness of certain forms of social competence.

5) The negative values toward the handicapped are learned in childhood by the handicapped, who accept and incorporate these values. This results in loss of self-esteem.

Studies of reactions and behavior that occur in response to initially meeting a person with a handicap have led me to develop the concept of "violation of expectation."

VIOLATION OF EXPECTATION

During the process of socialization we develop an increasingly complex set of expectations about the physical appearance of people, their dress, manner, speech, movement, and behavior. We are accustomed to some variability around these normative expectations. If, however, we encounter someone whose appearance, manner, or behavior exceeds the variability of our expectations, we respond with emotional arousal, anxiety, and fear. Such responses may well have been important for survival in our early ancestors. Today, responses to this violation of expectation may well be manifested in the kinds of behavior that occur in the reactions to a person with a handicap, the handicap appearing to constitute a violation of expectation. The responses to a violation of expectation can have serious interpersonal consequences for the person who caused the violation.

A number of questions and hypotheses are provoked by this concept. For example:

1) Norms and variations of expectations for appearance, manner, and behavior are based on the experiences of the individual. This would suggest that the earlier in life and the broader the range of people the individual has experienced, the less will be the likelihood of a violation of expectation. The more people who differ markedly in appearance, intelligence, and behavior are segregated and put away from our society, the more likely it is they will violate one's expectations.

2) If a person, on first meeting another, causes a violation of the other's expectations, the other person will, if there is continued interpersonal contact, become accustomed to what initially caused the violation of expectation, and the response of anxiety and fear will diminish and disappear. The more extreme the characteristic that caused the violation of expectation, the longer will be the exposure needed to diminish the anxiety and fear responses in others.

3) People appear largely unaware of the process of violation of expectation and the kinds of stimuli which will, for them, cause a violation of expectation. Further, they appear unaware of how their behavior may hurt those people who caused the violation. If people can gain awareness and understanding of what violates their expectations and what are the consequences of their resultant behavior, they will be less affected by the violation of expectation and broaden the variability they can accept around their normative expectations.

4) If a person can learn not to be upset by a characteristic that initially caused a violation of his expectations, will he be affected when a third party is present, and will he manifest different behavior caused by the violation of expectation of that third party?

5) For those persons whose appearance, manner, or behavior violates the expectations of others, awareness of the characteristic reactions of others may suggest ways of reducing the impact of the violation and of enabling the reactor to more quickly get over the effects of a violation.

A review of studies of more enduring interpersonal relations may partially answer some of the questions raised by considering the concept of violation of expectation.

Sociopsychologic Experiments

Kleck [27] carried out an experiment which differed from the studies we have reported in that the purpose of the interaction between nonhandicapped and handicapped persons was task oriented rather than a "get acquainted" social orientation. He also extended the time duration of the interpersonal relationship and used 2 separate interactions instead of 1. Subjects were given the task of training 2 persons (confederates of the experimenter) in origamy, a Japanese paper-folding skill. Neither confederate was handicapped, but they alternately simulated the role of a person with a left leg amputation. The roles alternated, but the same role was always used with a particular subject. In session I the subjects were taught origamy by the experimenter. In session II subjects then taught the origamy to a "handicapped" and a nonhandicapped confederate for 20 min. The subject continued teaching the confederates at session III, at a later time. The results showed that subjects who interacted with the "disabled" confederate formed more positive impressions of them than subjects did with nondisabled confederates. However, subjects did not come as close physically to their handicapped trainees as did subjects teaching nondisabled. As interaction time increased, both these behavioral tendencies diminished, and the author suggests that as subjects accumulated experience with the disabled the tendency to avoid proximate interaction was reduced.

Langer et al [28] proposed the hypothesis that avoidance is mediated by conflict over a desire to stare at novel stimuli and a desire to avoid the negative consequences that accompany staring when the novelty stimulus is another person. They predicted that the discomfort experienced in an initial social encounter between a handicapped and a nonhandicapped person stems from the discomfort of this conflict rather than from disparaging attitudes toward the handicapped. To test the hypothesis, they carried out an experiment where subjects entered a room, were given a chair and asked to sit down beside a handicapped person who was a confederate of the experimenter. However, before they entered the room, half the subjects viewed the handicapped person through a one-way mirror. The other subjects had no prior visual exposure. The degree of discomfort subjects felt was measured by the distance from the handicapped confederate that subjects placed their chairs. Subjects who had prior visual experience sat closer to the "novel" confederate who was physically handicapped than subjects with no prior visual exposure. There was also a tendency toward more favorable evaluation of the handicapped confederate when there had been previous visual access.

Interviewing Handicapped Persons

Davis [23] has reported that after the initial social encounter in which the physically handicapped are given fictional or surface acceptance, there is a second stage in the relationship which one informant described as "breaking through." "What takes place essentially is a redefinitional process in which the handicapped person projects images, attitudes and concepts of self which encourage the normal to identify with him (ie take his role) in terms other than those associated with imputations of deviance." This process is described by a handicapped person, ". . . and then as the relationship develops they don't see the handicap. It doesn't exist anymore. And that's the point that you as a handicapped individual become sensitive to. You know after talking with someone for a while that they don't see the handicap anymore. That's when you have broken through."

The final stage identified by Davis is when the person without a handicap relates to the personal qualities of the handicapped person but is also able to keep in mind the existence of the impairment and respond appropriately when the impairment restricts the handicapped person.

SOCIOMETRIC STUDIES

Sociometry has been used to study long-term social relationships of handicapped children in different settings. Force, and Centers and Centers [29, 30] studied handicapped children in classrooms with nonhandicapped children. The studies concluded that the handicapped children were less often chosen as friends, playmates, and workmates and most often chosen as least liked. In a summer camp for children attended by equal numbers of handicapped and nonhandicapped, a sociometric study was made of boys after they had lived together for 2 weeks [31]:

> . . . the handicapped boys were somewhat disadvantaged compared to the nonhandicapped boys, but differences occurred only on some measures. More specifically the visibly handicapped boys were intermediate and the nonhandicapped boys were most preferred. While these were persistent tendencies, there were not powerful differences in all the measures used. It is important to note . . . some of the visibly handicapped boys received many positive choices in and out of cabin, and some nonhandicapped received many negative choices.

The Socialization of Handicapped Children

In order to fully examine the cumulative effects of disability over time, studies of the socialization of handicapped children can provide valuable information. For example, Shere [32] studied a series of twins, one of whom had cerebral palsy. She found the handicapped twin was given less responsibility, fewer limits were placed on his or her behavior, the parents were more tolerant of deviant behavior, and he or she was more indulged.

Young adults with cerebral palsy, when asked to talk about their experiences of upbringing referred to a number of ways in which their disability had been a hindrance. They resented their education being interrupted for sessions of physical therapy and being in segregated classes for the handicapped; they felt they had been sheltered to the point where they were unable to make mistakes with the valuable learning that follows making mistakes; in adolescence they had been treated as though they had no sexual feelings; insufficient demands were placed on them to take responsibility. In addition, they felt that agencies which provide services for the handicapped have conceptions of appropriate roles for the handicapped which unnecessarily restrict their development and opportunities. Further, they resented the emphasis on what was wrong with them and a de-emphasis on their skills and competences [33].

Reports of parents' experiences in bringing up a child with a physical handicap tend to be of cases where the child is severely handicapped. Parents' initial reactions to the disability have already been summarized. The primary initial reaction to the physical appearance of the child appears to pass within the first year of life, at which time their reactions turn to the overall needs of the child, but still with attention, often necessarily, on what is wrong with the child. This emphasis is often reinforced by physicians and physical therapists who are trained toward a pathologic view and how the pathology may be alleviated or cured. Parents continually face the problem of trying to socialize their child and at the same time deal with the functional impairment of the child. The problem is described in the conclusion of a study by Hewett et al [34] of 180 mothers of children with cerebral palsy that their

> ... effort to 'treat the child as normal' has to be realistically related to the extent to which he is capable of behaving (and reacting to their behavior) like an unhandicapped child.... The parents and later the child himself must walk a tight-rope between acceptance of the fact that he is different from other children and insistence that he should be like them in as many ways as possible. If they emphasize his differences, continually 'making allowances' for his disability and learn a habit of helping and shielding, they may be branded 'overprotective'; if they minimize his handicap, treat him as an ordinary member of the family and speak with the optimism of his mental attainments of physical prospects, they may be judged to have 'failed' to accept the situation.

Parents also have to develop strategies for dealing with people who, in their initial encounters with the child, exhibit behaviors we have described earlier. Finally they have to deal with caring for the extra needs created by the handicap, together with seeking services which are often fragmented, only sometimes available, time consuming, and sometimes exhausting and frustrating to seek out and utilize. A difficult dilemma for the parents is that the additional time and energy required for the child with a handicap takes away from the time and attention that can be given the sibs and may lead to interpersonal tensions and problems for the family. The parents may well be aware of the needs of the handicapped child for companionship and social experience with peers, but if the impairment is severe, parents may be at a loss as to how to help the child obtain these experiences.

Observational Studies

Barker and Wright [35] observed the behavior of children with and without disabilities in naturally occurring situations in and outside the home using an ecologic perspective. They did not find a difference between disabled and non-disabled in the frequency of episodes ending with attainment or nonattainment, success or failure, and gratification or frustration.

Schoggen [36] observed matched pairs of children with and without a disability in the settings of home and classroom. He found little evidence in support of differential treatment and found that the handicap was generally disregarded in the behavior observed.

Institutions and Their Influence on Interpersonal Relations Between Those With and Without Disabilities

Institutions, created and maintained by our society, influence, sometimes profoundly, the attitudes and behavior toward the physically handicapped. The creation of special facilities for the handicapped for education, residential care, sheltered workshops, and recreation segregates the handicapped and reduces the opportunities for those who are not handicapped to meet and get to know those who are. Further, segregation occurs as the consequence of having public transportation, buildings, and toilets with obstacles such as steps and narrow doors which effectively bar persons with certain handicaps from using the facilities. Residential institutions have frequently been placed in isolated areas away from population centers, effectively cutting off the residents from social relationships formed prior to entry to the institution. Isolation of the institutions also influences the staff selection, and in many instances exacerbates the problem of staff turnover. The more those with physical handicaps are segregated and "put away," the more likely it is that their social relationships will be restricted and their opportunities limited for developing the kinds of social skills required in everyday life. This segregation is part of a broader set of social forces which clusters persons into patterns of living where those with like characteristics, such as age, color, and income, interact and avoid those with dissimilar characteristics. Institutions and agencies for the handicapped develop their own needs for survival and for stability of staff, and those needs can be in conflict with the needs of those they serve creating opposition to change and opposition to closing the institution, even when it is clear that this is in the best interest of those served by the institution [37].

EVALUATING THE RESULTS OF RESEARCH

The generalizations listed earlier and the speculation prompted by previous research were made with the recognition that it is necessary to be cautious and to consider the limitations imposed by the research methods employed. Some of the attitude studies reflect methodologic sophistication in developing scales of positive-negative attitudes toward the disabled and of social distance measures. Little attention, however, has been given to the stimuli used to elicit attitudes. The verbal label focuses exclusive attention on a handicap and ignores everything else about the person. Further, in addition to words having a denotative or descriptive function, words may also have connotative, implied, or suggestive meanings which include emotion or affect. Words, such as disabled, blind, amputee, may contain cues as to how the subject should react emotionally and influence his response.

For these reasons, it is necessary to be cautious in making inferences from the results about how people will react in an actual interpersonal situation with a handicapped person.

To avoid some of the difficulties and limitations of verbal stimuli used in attitude research, Richardson and his colleagues [38] examined initial reactions to disability by using visual cues of disability which included drawings of disabled and nondisabled children. The pictures avoid the problem of the connotation of words, and they portray the stimulus of a disability in the context of the visual representation of a child of a given age, dress, facial characteristics, color, and sex. Again, however, findings do not tell us the extent to which reactions to pictures predict behavior in interpersonal settings. The drawings show a child divorced from any social context or setting, and do not include many of the cues used in interpersonal evaluation such as movement, gesture, speech, and behavior.

In the sociopsychologic studies of interpersonal behavior, the requirements of experimental design influence both the questions asked and the procedures for securing evidence on which to base answers. The requirement of holding all but the experimental variable constant tempts the investigator to study only initial encounters. It is easier to hold constant the starting point of the social relationship if it is a first meeting. Further, the shorter the meeting the easier it is to hold constant the behavior of the confederate, who in most experiments plays dual roles of persons appearing as handicapped and as not handicapped. Unless the meeting is relatively short and superficial in nature, the behavior of the confederate becomes influenced by the subjects' behavior and confounds the study design. To test hypotheses, the behavior of a set of subjects is measured, and the mean differences and standard deviations of scores of behavior are used to determine the statistical significance of the differences found. The results are of general tendencies, and the individual variability of subjects tends to be overlooked.

Using a confederate who can give the appearance of being both handicapped and not handicapped restricts the kinds of handicap which can be simulated. Kleck and his colleagues used a wheelchair and the appearance of an amputation below the knee. Katz et al used a confederate sitting in a wheelchair. Langer et al used the presence or absence of a leg brace. Experiments share what appears to be the common tendency to get preoccupied with the presence or absence of the handicap and pay little attention to the characteristics of the confederate, the nature of the interpersonal relationship, or the setting in which the social encounter occurs, other than trying to hold them constant. Yet it is most likely that the extent to which a physical handicap influences even the initial encounter may depend to a considerable extent on the social and physical context of the encounter, together with the expectations of the subjects. If we are to get past learning that it is socially disadvantageous to be physically handicapped, we need to assess which factors can influence the extent to which the handicap is a salient factor in the social relationship and which other characteristics may increase or decrease the influence of the handicap. An encounter between strangers is a setting in which we have good reason to believe cues of physical appearance predominate, because until some interpersonal behavior takes place the wide range of other cues used in interpersonal evaluations have not been presented. What these nonappearance cues are and at what point they become salient are issues of major importance. Further, it is reasonable to suggest that with increasing interpersonal experience the salience of the physical handicap will diminish.

Data obtained from interviews with persons who are physically handicapped, or autobiographies of the handicapped, must also be interpreted with caution. Interviews which look for the problems of persons with physical handicaps will tend to find them. Instances of problems are well documented and often dramatic and poignant. What these do not tell us, though, is the frequency of these happenings, whether they are recurrent, everyday experiences or relatively rare events, and what are the characteristics of the people with whom they experience difficulties. There may be a tendency to select unusually intelligent, sensitive informants who recognize behavior of which others may not be aware. The same difficulties exist in autobiographies where there are pressures to focus on problems and difficulties.

The sociometric method has the advantage that the questions asked omit any reference to physical disability, for example, "who do you play with most" or "who is your best friend." We must be careful not to assume, however, that the findings reported are based on the response to visual cues of disability. The evidence on which they base their evaluation may range from interpersonal behavior, skills, abilities, and visual cues other than disability such as size, build, facial characteristics, and physical prowess. In the study of Richardson et al [38] the boys were all asked the reasons why they made their choices. The responses did not include reference to handicap but predominately dealt with behaviors such as aggressiveness, getting the cabin group into trouble, exhibiting behavior expected of younger children, and selfishness. This of course does not mean that the visual cues of disability were not relevant because they were not reported. As was suggested earlier, a physical handicap may lead to a child having less varied and frequent interpersonal experiences and as a result, less social competence.

Studies which report the socialization experiences of young people with physical handicaps deal with the overall effects of living in a society. These experiences clearly go beyond the initial reactions of the people and initial social encounters which take up so much of the research literature. Their experiences also go beyond others' responses to their physical appearance, which is also a dominant theme in the research literature. What those other experiences are is not made explicit but would include the direct consequences of the impairment, the experiences related to any treatment and therapy, the extra forms of care they have been given in their day to day lives, the possible experience of pain associated with the handicap, and how their life course has been influenced by being placed in special institutions for the handicapped. Unfortunately it is difficult to generalize from the experiences reported because of the small number of cases used and the probability that there is bias in selecting the more articulate and intelligent. However, the socialization experiences that have been reported do provide one of the best sources of insight and questions for more systematic study. The same is true for reports of the parents' experiences. Most of the studies of parents deal with their experiences during the early years of bringing up their handicapped children and the difficult adaptations they have to make. There are fewer accounts from older parents who have lived with their handicapped children through early adulthood.

It is unfortunate that there have not been more direct observational studies of children with and without physical handicaps in on-going interpersonal situations such as mixed classes at school or in summer camps. Inferences from research findings suggest that children with physical handicaps may be less socially competent, and yet we know very little directly about how they behave.

What appears to emerge from this review is that the studies which come close to achieving the requirements for scientific research do so at the price of over simplification such that it is necessary to be very cautious in generalizing the results to the more complex overall life experiences of those who are handicapped. On the other hand, the studies which attempt to take into account the complexities of everyday life come up with generalizations from limited and possibly biased case selection. We have learned a lot, and to conclude this stocktaking, I would like to suggest some of the research questions and issues which need pursuit in the future.

1) Research should include more complex social situations, eg how the behavior in a stabilized social relationship between a handicapped and nonhandi-

capped person is influenced by the introduction of a stranger or someone known to one or both parties.

2) More attention is needed on the variation which occurs in the distortion of behavior when a nonhandicapped person first meets a physically handicapped person. Also, we need to learn which factors influence the extent to which a person changes his or her behavior in an initial meeting with a handicapped person. This question was examined in attitude research but has been largely ignored in studies of interpersonal behavior. For example, in studying values toward handicap, Richardson [11] hypothesized that children whose individual values toward handicaps are similar to the group value will, when free to choose from a mixed group of peers with and without handicaps, choose as best friend someone who is not handicapped; whereas children whose values are atypical of the group value will choose someone who is handicapped. For children without handicaps the hypothesis was confirmed when choices were made soon after the group assembled for a 3-week camp, but not after they had been together for 2 weeks.

3) The effect of handicap on behavior has been studied under conditions where other factors which may influence interpersonal behavior have been held constant. It would be valuable now to begin systematically varying other factors to determine the extent to which changes in behavior toward the handicap are associated with other characteristics of the handicapped person, and the social and physical context in which the social interaction occurs, eg there is good evidence that interpersonal behavior is influenced by how good looking or ugly a person appears to another. What will be the differences in behavior exhibited toward a handicapped person who is good looking and toward one who is ugly? At a more complex level a multivariate design could examine combinations of different characteristics of a person, varying characteristics such as cues of movement, role, nature of the interpersonal task (eg socially or work oriented) degree of social and intellectual skill, skin color, etc.

4) There is some evidence that prior experience with persons who have a similar handicap reduces the degree to which a nonhandicapped person changes his behavior when meeting a handicapped person. Further studies are needed to confirm or contradict the evidence.

5) Various studies suggest that the proportion of majority and minority members within a group will have considerable effect on the interpersonal behavior between the majority and minority group members. For example, in colleges which have been exclusively for men and then change to coeducational, college administrators have suggested that until women represent between one-third to one-half of the student body they will be in a disadvantageous position. In schools, physically handicapped children are characteristically in segregated

classes, or, alternatively, they are in classes where they are the only ones with a handicap. Both these arrangements may be detrimental to the social development of the handicapped child. Summer-camp programs may provide unusually good opportunities for studies of different proportional mixes of handicapped and nonhandicapped children in the primary social group of the tent or cabin.

6) Despite what is known about interpersonal relations between handicapped and nonhandicapped, little attempt has been made in the education of children to teach understanding or appreciation of individual differences, to discuss questions dealing with differences in race, intelligence, wealth, physical handicap, and behavioral disturbance. It is even more surprising that educational authorities have not been concerned about these questions when, for whatever reason, they segregate various categories of children in special classes and thereby deprive those children without handicaps of the opportunity to get to know handicapped children. From discussions on these issues with 8–10-year-old children we have found that children are eager to discuss these questions. It is likely that they may bring up such issues with adults, but, because adults feel uncomfortable, embarrassed, and anxious when confronted with these discussions, they turn away the questions, and children learn these things are not "suitable" topics for discussion. How one gives childen an understanding and concern for individual differences and how one can help prepare them for satisfactory interpersonal relationships are questions where sensitive and wise pilot investigation is sorely needed. Such studies need to consider both content and method of teaching. Pieper [39] emphasized the need for special courses for teachers on the nature of handicap and the need to reach the children themselves. With the growing emphasis on mainstreaming, the early development of children's understanding of individual differences and provision of opportunities to develop interpersonal skills become urgent issues for research.

7) We need to learn more about the sources from which children derive their early learning about physical handicaps.

8) Research is needed to determine whether preparation for a social relationship with a handicapped person can relieve some of the difficulties reported in initial encounters. So far most studies have been designed so that the handicapped confederate is sprung on the subject without any warning. The only exception is the study of Langer et al who showed that prior visual exposure reduced the amount of behavior change in subjects' initial interaction with the handicapped. Preparation might be in the form of a discussion of what has been reviewed in this paper and the nature of cues used in interpersonal evaluation. Role playing might be useful in which subjects take the role of a handicapped or a nonhandicapped person in interpersonal relationships. Persons who are handicapped might play an effective part in such discussions.

At a very different level of interpersonal relationships, what forms of discussion with parents of a handicapped infant can be helpful to the parents? Research is needed both in the content of preparatory sessions and the methods to be used.

9) The review has shown that handicap creates barriers to normal social intercourse. There is anecdotal evidence of strategies used by handicapped persons to facilitate overcoming these barriers. Research is needed to cumulate information about these strategies and experiments conducted on their effectiveness. Such information would be invaluable to those who are handicapped.

10) There is evidence to suggest the handicapped child greatly needs a high level of social competence to overcome the initial barriers created by the handicap and assist "breaking through." Yet the handicapped child may well be deprived of many of the social experiences necessary for developing social competence, especially with peers. If these points are granted then there appears to be an important need to train handicapped children to avoid behaviors which lead to negative evaluation by peers and to develop social skills which are positively evaluated by peers. A prerequisite for training is research to learn what is considered social competence by children of different ages. More generally, we need to learn what are considered desirable personal characteristics among children and how these may vary in subcultures. For example, we observed a grossly obese girl at a summer camp who initially was at a major social disadvantage because of her obesity. One of the counselors, who was a musician, found out the girl was a talented blues singer. The girl and the counselor rehearsed and then gave a performance at a meal where all the children were gathered. She was given a standing ovation, and there appeared to be a major change in children's behavior toward her for the remainder of camp.

11) There appears to be wide variability in the competence of children with comparable handicaps to get along with their peers. By careful examination of their life histories and the factors which influenced their socialization we may obtain clues to account for the differences. We may then use the findings to determine whether there are factors which have implications for the socialization and training of handicapped children.

No further research is needed to show that it is socially disadvantageous to be physically handicapped in initial social encounters. The literature suggests that the initial social disadvantage is powerful and pervasive, but the research methods used and the nature of the inferences made from the evidence may have exaggerated the problems. Insufficient attention has been given to considering whether statistically significant differences are also socially significant differences. In more extended social relationships, whether the person with a physical handicap continues to be at a social disadvantage is less clear. Some studies show differences and others do not. In future research we need more direct studies of behavior in which there is less need to make large inferential jumps in interpreting results.

ACKNOWLEDGMENTS

The author is grateful to Helene Koller for her critical and constructive comments on drafts of this paper and her editorial assistance; also to the Foundation for Child Development for financial support.

REFERENCES

1. Barker, R. G., Wright, B. A., Meyerson, L., and Gonick, M.: "Adjustment to Physical Handicap and Illness: A Survey of the Social Psychology of Physique and Disability." New York: Social Science Research Council, 1953.
2. Yuker, H. E., Block, J. R., and Younng, J. H.: "The Measurement of Attitudes Toward Disabled Persons." Albertson, New York: Human Resources Center, 1966.
3. Siller, J., Ferguson, L., Vann, D. H., and Holland, B.: "Structure of Attitudes Toward the Physically Disabled." New York: New York University School of Education, 1967.
4. Richardson, S. A., Goodman, N., Hastorf, A. H., and Dornbush, S. M.: Cultural uniformity in reaction to physical disabilities. Am. Sociol. Rev. 26:241–247, 1961.
5. Goodman, N., Richardson, S. A., Dornbush, S. M., and Hastorf, A. H.: Variant reactions to physical disabilities. Am. Sociol. Rev. 28:429–435, 1963.
6. Richardson, S. A., and Royce, J.: Race and physical handicap in children's preference for other children. Child Dev. 39:467–480, 1968.
7. Richardson, S. A., and Emerson, P.: Race and physical handicap in children's preference for other children: A replication in a Southern city. Hum. Relations 23:31–36, 1970.
8. Richardson, S. A.: Age and sex differences in values toward physical handicaps. J. Health and Soc. Behav. 11:207–214, 1970.
9. Richardson, S. A.: Handicap, appearance and stigma. J. Soc. Sci. Med. 5:621–628, 1971.
10. Richardson, S. A., and Green, A.: When is black beautiful? Coloured and white children's reactions to skin colour. Br. J. Educ. Psychol. 41:62–69, 1971.
11. Richardson, S. A.: Children's values and friendships: A study of physical disability. J. Health Soc. Behav. 12:253–258, 1971.
12. Richardson, S. A., and Friedman, M. J.: Social factors related to children's accuracy in learning peer group values towards handicaps. Hum. Relations 26:77–87, 1972.
13. Baskin, B. H.: The handicapped child in children's literature themes, patterns and stereotypes. The English Record 26:91–99, 1974.
14. Kagan, J., Henker, B. A., Hen-Tov, A., Levine, J., and Lewis, M.: Infants' differential reactions to familiar and distorted faces. Child Dev. 37(3):518–532, 1966.
15. Kleck, R., Ono, H., and Hastorf, A. H.: The effects of physical deviance upon face-to-face interaction. Hum. Relations 19(4):425–436, 1966.
16. Kleck, R.: Physical stigma and nonverbal cues emitted in face-to-face interaction. Hum. Relations 21:19–28, 1968.
17. Kelley, H. H., Hastorf, A. H., Jones, E. E., Thibaut, J. W., and Usdane, W. M.: Some implications of social psychological theory for research on the handicapped. In Lofquist, L. H. (ed.): "Psychological Research and Rehabilitation." Report of a conference of the American Psychological Association, Miami Beach, 1960, pp. 172–204.
18. Katz, I., Glass, D. C., Lucido, D. J., and Farber, J. E.: Ambivalence, guilt, and the denigration of a physically handicapped victim. (Unpublished.)

19. Strasser, H., and Sievert, G.: Some psycho-social aspects of ectromelia: A preliminary report of a research study. In Swinyard, C. A. (ed.): "Proceedings of a Conference on Human Limb Development and Maldevelopment with Special Reference to Experimental Teratogenesis and Medical Management of Limb Deficiencies." The Hague, Holland. New York: Association for the Aid of Crippled Children, 1969.
20. Drotar, D., Baskiewicz, B. A., Irvin, N., Kennell, J., and Klaus, M.: The adaptation of parents to the birth of an infant with a congenital malformation: A hypothetical model. Pediatrics 56:710–717, 1975.
21. Hunt, G. M.: Implications of the treatment of myelomeningocele for the child and his family. Lancet. 12:1308–1310, 1973.
22. Roskies, E.: "Abnormality and Normality." Ithaca and London: Cornell University Press, 1972.
23. Davis, F.: Deviance disavowal: The management of strained interaction by the visibly handicapped. Social Problems. 9(2):120–132, 1961.
24. Hathaway, K. B.: "The Little Locksmith." New York: Coward-McCann Press, 1943.
25. Viscardi, H.: "A Man's Stature." New York: John Day, 1952.
26. MacGregor, F. C., Abel, T. M., Bryt, A., Lauer, E., and Weissmann, S.: "Facial Deformities and Plastic Surgery – A Psychosocial Study." Springfield: Charles C Thomas, 1953.
27. Kleck, R.: Physical stigma and task oriented interactions. Hum. Relations 22:53–59, 1969.
28. Langer, E. J., Taylor, S., Fiske, S., and Chanowitz, B.: Stigma, staring and discomfort. J. Exp. Soc. Psychol. (In press.)
29. Force, D. G.: Social status of physically handicapped children. Except. Child. 23:104–107, 1956.
30. Centers, L., and Centers, R.: Peer group attitudes toward the amputee child. J. Soc. Psychol. 61:127–132, 1963.
31. Kleck, R., Richardson, S. A., and Ronald, L.: Physical appearance cues and interpersonal attraction in children. Child Dev. 45:305–310, 1974.
32. Shere, M. D.: Socio-emotional factors in the family of twins with cerebral palsy. Except. Child. 22:196–199, 206–208, 1956.
33. Richardson, S. A.: People with cerebral palsy talk for themselves. Dev. Med. Child Neurol. 14:524–535, 1972.
34. Hewett, S., Newsom, J., and Newsom, E.: "The Family and the Handicapped Child: A Study of Cerebral Palsied Children in Their Homes." London: George Allen & Unwin, 1970.
35. Barker, R. G., and Wright, H. F.: "Midwest and its Children: The Psychological Ecology of an American Town." Evanston, Ill.: Peterson, 1955.
36. Schoggen, P.: Observed behavior of mothers and teachers toward children with physical disabilities in natural settings. (Unpublished.)
37. Ohlin, L. E.: Reforming programs for youth in trouble. In Begab, M. J. and Richardson, S. A. (eds.): "The Mentally Retarded and Society." Baltimore, London, Tokyo: University Park Press, 1974.
38. Richardson, S. A., Ronald, L., and Kleck, R.: The social status of handicapped and non-handicapped boys living together. J. Spec. Ed. 8:143–152, 1974.
39. Pieper, E.: Preparing children for a handicapped classmate. The Instructor 84:128–129, 1974.

Research on Families With Handicapped Children — An Aid or an Impediment to Understanding?

Sheila Hewett, PhD

Our aim here is to increase understanding of the problems of the handicapped. In the search for understanding, social workers, doctors, or any other practitioners who are involved with handicapped children and their families may well turn, from time to time, to the reports of research which has been carried out in their field. The research worker, who in his own way is also concerned to help the handicapped, must do the same before he carries out his own studies. The same problem will immediately confront them all. If they read more than one book or paper they will discover confusing differences in the ways in which studies have been conducted and even more confusion and conflict in the results.

This paper will discuss some of the problems presented by research on the families of children who suffer from cerebral palsy or mental retardation. It is possible to look at only a few examples, both American and British, out of an enormous literature on these topics.

Some of the earliest surveys of cerebral-palsied children in Britain were undertaken mainly to establish the prevalence of the condition and to describe the characteristics of its sufferers. Dunsdon [1] and Schonell [2], in the 1950s, both carried out wide surveys; in addition to their main findings they commented that the guilty feelings of parents caused them to overprotect their children to the detriment of their development. They did not describe in sufficient detail the methods they had used in order to establish this fact, so that their approach could not be replicated. It is far from clear in these studies what kinds of behavior count as being overprotective. However, even when apparently objective criteria are used in making such judgments, there is no guarantee that the judgments themselves will be consistently objective. Beatrice Wright [3] points this out and lists criteria which she has reproduced from the often-quoted study by Shere [4] of 30 pairs of twins, one of each pair being cerebral-palsied. Ten signs of overprotectiveness are quoted, and 12 deleterious effects of such overprotection in terms of the child's behavior are described. However, the behavior in both lists can occur in any family for a variety of reasons at one time or another. The circumstances in which they become pathologic need clarification. For instance, to say that a child "may like to read rather than play," that "he may have temper tantrums" (to quote only 2 of the behaviors listed as indicative that the child has been overprotected) is not very informative. Children whose parents are not considered overprotective toward them may well exhibit similar behaviors from time to time. At what point does such behavior become abnormal and undesirable? As Wright points out, "the judgment as to whether the child is being overprotected, however, depends on who is doing the evaluating." In addition to this, whether he is handicapped or not, a child's emotional needs may be different from those of his brothers and sisters. As the Newsons' [5] study of normal children shows, a child may well insist on more indulgence from his mother than she herself feels is appropriate. In this way, he may ensure that his needs are met even when they do not conform to the pattern considered desirable in his cultural setting.

When attempts are made to verify the alleged effects of adverse parental attitudes on the handicapped children concerned, the results can still be conflicting. Martorana [6] in 1954 subjected 32 handicapped and 32 normal children, matched for age and intelligence, to objective and projective tests. He also investigated the attitudes of their mothers. He found that scores on attitude scales did not differ significantly for the 2 groups of mothers and concluded that "poor parent-child relationships and maladjustment in the crippled appeared to be due mainly to the child's handicaps." A similar finding is reported by Block [7] who used 20 "spastics" and 18 "athetoids," randomly selected from out-patient departments and schools in New York City. Mallison [8], on the other hand, using case-study methods to explore similar problems, came to the opposite conclusion that the emotional adjustment of handicapped children was dependent more upon the attitudes of their mothers than on the severity of their handicaps.

Miller [9], studying children who had been referred to a child-guidance clinic, compared those known to be cerebral-palsied with the nonhandicapped and found considerable similarity between the behavior problems of the 2 groups. Among the cerebral-palsied, the least handicapped had the most serious emotional difficulties, and this was attributed to differences in parental attitudes — parents found it harder to accept the limitations of near normality than the obvious handicaps of severe disability.

The study by Miller made use of a highly selected sample of children, ie those referred to a child-guidance clinic, and it may be that the emphasis on the emotional problems of the cerebral-palsied and their families is to a certain extent attributable to the fact that much of the evidence has been garnered from similar samples in clinical situations. This may also account in some measure for the conflicting evidence. The problem is well discussed by Kelman [10] in a paper which also questions the appropriateness of some current models of family function which emphasize what he calls "intra-familial psychological variables" at the expense of the family's sociologic functions.

It is perhaps from clinical situations that the concept of the handicapped family has evolved. The concept is presented and evidence is offered to establish its validity by Goldie [11], a psychiatrist, who suggests that it is disastrous to consider the child in isolation from his family and to ignore the adaptations the family has had to make ever since the handicap has been known to them, possibly right from birth. He also suggests that physicians "should be aware of the psychologic implications (of handicap) and should ensure that where necessary psychiatric care should start as soon as possible." Another psychiatrist, A. I. Roith [12], however, talks of "the myth of parental attitudes" and suggests that "much of what has been published is purely anecdotal in character or else based on mere impressions." Roith was concerned with the parents of mentally retarded children and his paper is of particular interest because he attempted to test the assumptions with which he had originally approached his work as a clinician, using research methods to do so. A study of the literature on handicap, combined with personal experience of speakers at a number of meetings concerning the mentally subnormal, had led him to believe that he would observe many adverse attitudes in parents of subnormal children, including a good deal of guilt. In practice, this did not happen with the families referred to him. To see whether things were the same with others he had not met, he sent a postal questionnaire to all parents of patients in Monyhull Hospital, Birmingham, 120 in all. He concluded from the replies given on the returned questionnaires that the problems had been exaggerated. However, the result was not as reliable as one would wish, since, as so often happens with postal questionnaires, the response rate was poor, 60% only being returned.

Returning to the concept of the handicapped family, which is currently very much in use in Britain, some basis for discussing how far and in what ways such a family differs from the nonhandicapped family has to be found if the concept is to be useful. The 3 case studies offered by Goldie in the above-mentioned paper were of families where the child had been referred for psychiatric treatment, a fact which of itself makes them atypical, since the vast majority of handicapped children are not referred to psychiatric clinics in the UK.

A broader case study approach has been taken recently in Britain by Kew [3]. He has analyzed the reports made by case workers on more than 500 families with a handicapped child referred to a voluntary organization in the London area and from these and to a small extent from his own case load, he has analyzed the problems experienced by the sibs of the handicapped children. Again, it is unusual for families to be regularly visited by case workers — this happens, as Kew acknowledges, because they have what he calls psychosocial problems, and the main concern of the agency in his study is with such problems. He acknowledges too that such a study can give no perspective on the extent of problems in families with handicapped children generally, but feels that perspective is less important than the recognition of families with a handicapped child as handicapped families.

Other researchers, unlike Kew, consider that it is essential to see how much the family interactions of the handicapped differ from those of normal children and their parents. One study which included a control group was carried out by Boles [14], who compared 60 mothers of cerebral-palsied children with 60 mothers who had no handicapped children. The mothers were matched on 10 variables. They completed self-administered attitude questionnaires which had been devised specifically for the project. On their replies, Boles based his conclusion that the mothers of the cerebral-palsied children were more overprotective than the controls and had more marital conflicts but that both groups felt considerable guilt and both were anxious and rejecting, a very interesting finding, especially when considered in the light of Erikson's [15] comment in 1963 that the rejecting mother appeared to be an occupational prejudice among psychiatrists.

Boles' work, although interesting, does not really make the move away from assessing mothers' attitudes, albeit in a scientifically controlled way, to the study of the family itself that an appraisal of the concept of the handicapped family requires. An early study by Larson [16] of the experience of 135 young children with a variety of physical handicaps, including 74 with cerebral palsy, moved some way toward this. He interviewed the parents of the handicapped children and of 135 physically normal children, using an interview schedule that covered 4 broad areas of experiences provided for children within the family setting. These 4 areas concern what Larson calls: 1) socialization — opportunities for interaction with other children and with adults; 2) recognition — the ways in which parents acknowledge the child as a person by giving him books, a room of his own, and personal attention; 3) outside experiences — trips to shops, museums, parks, etc; 4) knowledge and experience — songs and nursery rhymes known, responsibility for personal hygiene, for pets, and many similar items. He found that the handicapped children were at a disadvantage in all areas and that parents had not apparently been at pains to compensate them for the restrictions imposed by their disabilities, possibly because they were not aware of the importance of doing so. This is a useful approach because it deals with the specific activities by means of which the family meets the child's needs and which provide the framework within which he can develop. It would have been even more useful if the activities of the handicapped children's normal brothers and sisters had also been investigated. It would then have been clearer how the family itself was affected by the presence of the handicap. One cannot help wondering whether the handicapped children were simply excluded from a number of excursions and privileges or whether the whole family's activities were curtailed. It is not clear from Larson's report whether any of the physically handicapped children were also mentally retarded. Since some were cerebral-palsied and others were epileptic, this is a possibility. If it were so, it might help to account for the somewhat puzzling finding that while 95% of the "normal" group were said to be familiar with the story of Goldilocks and the 3 bears, only 55% of the "handicapped" group knew this story. It is hard to conceive of the circumstances in which a child with a purely physical handicap is deliberately excluded from storytelling sessions. One can only speculate — had prolonged hospitalization been a crucial factor in the deprivation of experience? Similarly, there seems to be no common sense reason why a child with polio or with only one arm, should be less aware of "the sources of common food stuffs" than any other child. One would like to know a good deal more about these children and to know whether particular gaps in experience were handicap-specific or not.

Larson's finding does not seem to be very consistent with Boles' observation that mothers can become so preoccupied with the needs of their cerebral-palsied children that the needs of the normal children are neglected. If they are indeed so preoccupied, one would expect to find that the handicapped children's needs were adequately met, possibly at the expense of any normal children in the family. This was the conclusion reached by Shere [4], who stated that "the condition of cerebral palsy can be more harmful to the social and emotional development of the nonhandicapped child than to his twin who has cerebral palsy."

Conflicting research results confuse the issue in other respects as well. Cockburn [17], for example, like Boles, found that parents were unrealistic about their children's future possibilities, but where Cockburn found that they became more realistic as the children grew older, Boles found the reverse to be true of his samples. Again, Boles found evidence of increased marital conflict where there was a cerebral-palsied child, whereas Schaffer [18] found that 13 of his sample of 30 families having a cerebral-palsied child exhibited a pathologic degree of parental and familial solidarity — the so-called too-cohesive familes. Schaffer used interviews and time-sampling to study these families and devised an operational definition of family cohesiveness. This involved the expression of "time spent together" by family members as a percentage of time they could have spent together, allowing for normal school and work hours. The families thus categorized as too-cohesive were seen by Schaffer as being potentially very unstable. All their interests and interfamilial relationships were channeled via a single concern, ie the child and his handicap. Schaffer's judgment of the nature of the increased involvement of the 13 too-cohesive families goes beyond the evidence of the increased involvement itself. He suggests, for example, that the father's involvement was greater than would have been "culturally expected," but one wonders about the accuracy of cultural expectations. The sample he saw was a fairly homogeneous, Scottish working-class group. Research experience in Nottingham has shown that some of the stereotypes of working-class attitudes and behavior do not hold in that city, particularly with reference to the father's role in bringing up the children. Many of Nottingham's working-class fathers now stay at home and give the baby his bottle instead of spending all their spare time at the "local." Perhaps changes are taking place in Scotland, as well.

Even more fundamental to the problem of judging different patterns of family organization is the fact that there is no kind of family organization that can be immediately categorized as pathologic or unstable per se. As Elizabeth Bott [19] pointed out after studying 20 "ordinary" British families intensively, there is variation in the ways in which families function and meet the needs of each member.

Goldberg [20] drew similar conclusions as to the variety of family organizations that could be satisfactory for the family concerned from the normal families who formed the control group in a study concerned with psychosomatic illness. She says, "the most striking impression I carried away with me from the investigation was the great variety of ways in which people can relate to one another and be reasonably happy and how unlike the child guidance stereotype of the well-adjusted family these adaptations really were."

The studies discussed so far have mainly centered around cerebral palsy in children, but conflicting research results also confuse the issues in studies of mental retardation. Farber [21], for example, devised a scale for measuring "marital integration" and "sib role tension" in an attempt to measure the ways in which the presence of retarded children affected their families. He came to the conclusion that marital integration, as defined by his scale, remained the same whether mentally retarded girls were sent to institutions or stayed at home but that it was impaired when retarded boys were kept at home. Fowle [22] used the same scales but was unable to show similar differences in marital integration. She did, however, corroborate Farber's finding that sisters, especially older sisters, are more affected by dependent retarded children in the home than are brothers.

In England, Gath [23, 24] twice studied the brothers and sisters of children with Down syndrome. She used measures devised by Rutter [25] to assess the degree to which they showed disturbed behavior, compared with controls with no handicapped sibs. Rutter's scales are completed by parents and teachers. In Gath's first study, index and control children were matched on 7 variables, and the sibs of the handicapped children were not rated as showing disturbed behavior more often than the controls. In the second, less well-controlled study, Rutter's scales were used again and this time teacher, but not parents, reported disturbed behavior in sibs of index children significantly more often than in the controls. The percentages were very small (13% and 7%, respectively), and the finding seems less important in the light of Rutter's statement that his scales are for screening purposes, not diagnosis. If children rated as disturbed by either parent or teacher alone are subsequently examined by a psychiatrist, about half of them are likely to be seen to have no diagnosable psychiatric problems. However, if both parents and teachers rate behavior disturbance, 75% of these children are likely to have a diagnosable problem, but parent and teacher ratings do not often overlap. In Gath's second study, only one child was rated as disturbed by both parent and teacher. Gath suggests that explanations for difficult behavior lay in large family size, financial hardship, and parental pressure, rather than simply arising from the presence of a handicapped child. Rutter himself came to the conclusion that the most reliable method of obtaining information about children's behavior was to interview their parents.

These examples have been offered to illustrate how carefully research results must be studied and assessed. If casework studies alone are considered, the reader will tend to be convinced that all families with handicapped children are overwhelmed by emotional problems. The studies which have attempted to use rigorous scientific method in applying scales and controlling variables will leave the impression that the extent to which problems exist is not reliably measurable.

Surveys of samples which are representative of specified handicaps, particularly when careful interviewing techniques are used and when they can be continued longitudinally, offer the means both for discovering problems and for placing these problems in context and in perspective. At the same time, they allow proper description of the problems, so that their significance for the individuals who experience them is not minimized, even though they may occur in only a minority of families.

This was the method used by Hewett [26] to study the way cerebral-palsied children were brought up in the late 1960s, in the midlands of England. Few differences were reported by the mothers of the handicapped children, compared with mothers of normal children. In addition, there were striking similarities with the findings of Barsch [27] who carried out a similar but much larger comparative study, using interview methods among others, in the US at about the same time. When the East Midlands cerebral palsy method was used to study other populations, for example, by Carr [28] who studied children with Down syndrome, there was a remarkable consistency in findings that suggest that the mothers of handicapped children themselves are commendably successful in the majority of cases in coping with the undeniable difficulties they encounter. I am inclined to agree with Barsch when he says: "The general tendency to characterize parents of handicapped children as guilt-ridden, anxiety-laden, over-protective and rejecting beings is unfortunate. While it is true that such cases exist, the majority of parents are unduly stigmatised by this generalization."

Carr's study, which included matched control children and was longitudinal from 6 months to 4 years, is now being continued by Carr and Hewett, after a 7-year interval. Mothers have been interviewed and Rutter's scales used to test again their usefulness in indicating differences between sibs of the Down syndrome children and the sibs of their normal controls. It is only by patient replication and constant refinement of research techniques in the light of experience that progress can be made in the application of scientific method to the clarification of human problems.

In spite of the differences between research methods there are themes which appear consistently in all types of research findings, so that one feels convinced that they must have some general importance.

Broadly, 2 types of problems emerge over and over again. There are the practical problems which require money for their solution — these include the provision of attendance allowances, now paid to many parents in Britain; appliances; adaptations to homes; medical, educational, and social services of all kinds. These are still inadequate in the UK and will remain so for some time, given the present economic situation. The other kind of problem requires not money but thought, imagination, time, and effort on the part of individual workers. Since they cost nothing, they are or should be, more susceptible to solution than the others.

One such problem concerns all handicapped children and their families. Most systematic British studies show that parents themselves say repeatedly that they are not given enough information either about the child's condition or about ways of dealing with it at home. This problem starts when a diagnosis has to be communicated to the parents, and this can be either at birth or, as is so often the case with cerebral palsy and mental retardation, at any time during the first year of life when delayed development indicates that something is wrong. Evidence from studies where mothers have been asked their views on when and how to be told the diagnosis is summarized [29] in a short paper contributed to a symposium on this problem held in London in 1973. Considerable dissatisfaction was reported. Carr [30] in her study of children with Down syndrome, found that although 60% of mothers had been told within a month of the birth and 93% within 6 months, a third of them wished they had been told sooner. Half of those told within the first week would have like to have been told even sooner. They said that their questions to hospital staff were not answered or were parried by reassuring platitudes, or they were actually told lies about the babies. The earlier they were told, the more likely were mothers to be satisfied with how and when they were told. Clearly breaking such bad news to parents is a difficult task for medical and nursing staff. In British hospitals, where nursing staff are often forbidden to discuss matters with patients before the doctor in charge of the case has had time to do so, the nurses are forced to temporize and prevaricate when mothers ask them questions. Doctors may delay the telling, in some cases because they believe that it is harmful to the mother's relationship with the child to tell her "too soon," although there is no systematic evidence to support this view. They more often have little time for discussion and little skill in communicating with people who do not understand medical terminology. In some medical schools in Britain doctors in training are now being taught this essential skill by, for example, seeing on videotape recordings how they themselves have behaved when talking to "actress-patients" [31]. The initial telling of the parents that they have a handicapped child must be followed by the repeated offering of advice on management and information about the condition by any and all health care or social workers who may see the family subsequent to the birth. It has been shown by several researchers, but notably by Matheny and Vernick [32] in the US and by Bobath and Finnie [33] in the UK that counseling without comprehensible information and practical help is of little value. Matheny and Vernick particularly warn counselors that they may not do their work well if they concentrate too much on what they see as emotional aberrations in the parents. Psychotherapy is no substitute for knowledge or for help with caring for the child. Carr [34] too has described how well the parents of severely retarded children respond when they are taught to use behavior-modification techniques successfully with their children.

A second important problem is relevant to only a minority of handicapped children and their families, because it concerns the need to have the child cared for away from the family. In Britain, most handicapped children, even those who are both mentally and physically handicapped, are looked after at home. This is the wish and the achievement of the majority of parents. To give an example, 42 of the cerebral-palsied children who were studied by the author in 1965/66 were visited again in 1974 by another researcher when they were aged from 14 to 16 years old [35]. Of the children visited 80% were still at home. Only 8% (4 children) had been taken into residential care, and 3 of these were very severely handicapped. Their mothers were among 19 who had said at the earlier stage of the study that they thought residential care might become necessary later. Ten of these mothers still had their children at home and the remaining 5 children in this group had died. Wing [36], reporting in 1973 on 100 mentally retarded children aged between 0–14 years, found that 22% were in residential care and a further 14% of the mothers wanted such care for their children.

It is frequently suggested that wanting residential care indicates a rejecting attitude in the mother. However, when a study was made by the author [37] of children admitted for such care comparing them with similar children still at home, the results suggested that the mothers of the admitted children more often reported certain difficulties than the mothers of children still at home, eg that the child had slept badly, causing many disturbed nights, there was a poor relationship between mother and father, the sibs were having difficulties, and the parents had been given a hopeless prognosis for the child. The mothers of admitted children in the Wing [36] study gave somewhat similar accounts. Half the mothers in the Hewett study thought that no possible help could have kept the child at home and in almost all these cases the circumstances prior to admission were such that they were surely right — parental ill-health, gross hydrocephaly in the child, absence or loss of a parent. More than 80% of the mothers found it painful that the child was not living at home, even though their admission seemed unavoidable. In fact, the institutionalizing of the child had added new stresses to their existing problems, even if it had relieved the burden of actually caring for the child. This is not always understood by professionals, who see only the relief offered, not the distress. Mothers spoke of the guilt they felt at relinquishing the care of the child to strangers, of the distress at simply being a visitor to the child, the misery caused by the knowledge that subnormality hospitals are not the best places for children to live in. If community or, more accurately, family care comes to be even more widely the preferred care for the handicapped in the future, the stress on parents who are forced by circumstances to have their children admitted to residential care will be even greater. Professional workers who have contact with such mothers will have to guard against increasing their distress, which they could well do if they imply that the parents are rejecting or glad to be rid of their burdens. Hospital staff too, who criticize parents for not visiting their children enough should remember the comments of the parents who admitted that they visited infrequently. They said that when they saw the child they longed to bring him home, that his life in the hospital was a living death. It took them days to recover from seeing him and all the other children. None of the parents regarded the acceptance of residential care as a positive choice, made specifically for the welfare of the child. How different this situation is from the hospitalization of normal children for treatment. However, if the reforms in residential care which have been started continue, parents may come to see the acceptance of such care as having positive value for their child and more of them may then seek it. Professionals must then be aware of the conflicts of emotion that parents experience when taking such a decision and must help to relieve them of their sense of failure and loss. They must also be offered a positive relationship with the institutions which take over and deprive them of their parental responsibilities.

Above all, parents of handicapped children should not readily or lightly be categorized or stereotyped, either by regarding too seriously those reports which dwell only on problems or by allowing the general trends discovered by surveys to obscure individual differences. Each family is unique in its experience of handicap.

REFERENCES

1. Dunsdon, M. I.: "The Educability of Cerebral Palsied Children." National Foundation Education Research, London: Newnes, 1952.
2. Schonell, E.: "Educating Spastic Children." London: Oliver and Boyd, 1956.

3. Wright, B. A.: "Physical Disability – A Psychological Approach." New York: Harper & Row, 1960.
4. Shere, M. O.: An evaluation of the social and emotional development of the cerebral palsied twin. (Unpublished doctoral dissertation.) Michigan, Ann Arbor University Microfilms, publication no. 9140.
5. Newson, J., and Newson, E.: "Four Years Old in an Urban Community." London: Allen and Unwin, 1968.
6. Martorana, A. A.: A comparison of the personal, emotional, and family life of crippled and normal children. (Ph.D. thesis, 1954, University of Minnesota.)
7. Block, W. E.: Somatopsychological relationships in cerebral palsied children. In "Exceptional Children," vol. 22, 1955–56.
8. Mallinson, V.: "None Can Be Called Deformed." London: Heinemann, 1956.
9. Miller, E. A.: Cerebral palsied children and their parents. A study in child-parent relationships. Except. Child. 24:298–302, 1958.
10. Kelman, H. R.: The brain damaged child and his family. In Birch, H. G. (ed.): "Brain Damage in Children – The Biological and Social Aspects." Baltimore: Williams and Wilkins, 1964.
11. Goldie, L.: The psychiatry of the handicapped family. Dev. Med. Child Neurol. 8:456, 1966.
12. Roith, A. I.: The myth of parental attitudes. J. Ment. Subnorm. 9:51–54, 1963.
13. Kew, S.: "Handicap and Family Crisis. A Study of the Siblings of Handicapped Children." London: Pitman, 1975.
14. Boles, G.: Personality factors in mothers of cerebral palsied children. Genet. Psychol. Monogr. 59:159, 1959.
15. Erikson, E. H.: "Childhood and Society." New York: Norton; London: Hogarth, 1963.
16. Larson, L.: Preschool experiences of physically handicapped children. Except. Child. 24:310, 1958.
17. Cockburn, J. M.: In Henderson (ed.): "Cerebral Palsy in Childhood and Adolescence." Edinburgh and London: Livingstone, 1961.
18. Schaffer, H. R.: The too-cohesive family – a form of group pathology. Int. J. Soc. Psychiatry X:266–275, 1964.
19. Bott, E.: "Family and Social Network." London: Social Science Paperbacks, 1968.
20. Goldberg, E. M.: The normal family – myth and reality. In Younghusband, E. (ed.): "Social Work with Families." London: Allen and Unwin, 1965.
21. Farber, B.: Effects of a severely retarded child on family integration. Monogr. Soc. Res. Child. Dev. 2:24, 1959.
22. Fowle, C. M.: Effect of a severely retarded child on the family. Am. J. Ment. Defic. 73:468, 1968.
23. Gath, A.: The mental health of siblings of congenitally abnormal children. J. Child. Psychol. Psychiatry 13:211, 1972.
24. Gath, A.: The school age siblings of mongol children. Br. J. Psychiatry 123:161, 1973.
25. Rutter, M., Tizard, J., and Whitmore, K. (eds.): "Education, Health and Behaviour." London: Longmans, 1970.
26. Hewett, S. H.: "The Family and the Handicapped Child." London: Allen and Unwin, 1970.
27. Barsch, R. H.: "The Parent of the Handicapped Child." Springfield: Charles C Thomas, 1968.
28. Carr, J.: "Young Children with Down's Syndrome." London: Butterworths, 1975.
29. Hewett, S. H.: Telling the family. In Spain, B., and Wigley, G. (eds.): "Right From the Start." London: National Society Mentally Handicapped Children, 1975, pp. 23–27.

30. Carr, J.: Mongolism – telling the parents. Dev. Med. Child Neurol. 12:213, 1970.
31. Meadow, R., and Hewitt, C.: Teaching communication skills with the help of actresses and videotape. Br. J. Med. Educ. 6:317, 1972.
32. Matheny, A. P., and Vernick, J.: Parents of the mentally retarded child – emotionally overwhelmed or informationally deprived? J. Pediatr. 74:953, 1969.
33. Bobath, B., and Finnie, N. R.: Problems of communication between parents and staff in the treatment and management of children with cerebral palsy. Dev. Med. Child Neurol. 12:629, 1970.
34. Carr, J.: Behaviour modification (as applied to the severely retarded at Hilda Lewis House). In "Right From the Start," op. cit., pp. 91–95.
35. Venning, H.: Cerebral palsy in children – a longitudinal study assessing the development of functional abilities. (Unpublished dissertation.) University of Nottingham, 1975.
36. Wing, L.: Problems experienced by parents of children with severe mental retardation. In "Right From the Start," op. cit., pp. 33–36.
37. Hewett, S. H.: In "Occasional Papers in Mental Retardation." Papers 2, 3, and 4, Paper 3. London: Butterworth, 1972, pp. 59–101.

The Disabled Child at School: Special Needs and Special Provision

Elizabeth M. Anderson, MA, BSc, PhD

My main aim in this paper is to discuss the psychologic and social implications of developmental disabilities in relation to schooling. In this paper I shall talk mainly about preadolescent schoolchildren. Research suggests that there are clear differences between the functioning of disabled children with and without brain disorders — between, for example, children with cerebral palsy or with spina bifida and associated hydrocephalus on the one hand and children disabled by, let us say, congenital skeletal defects or muscular dystrophy on the other. The former, that is the brain disorder group, are much more likely to be retarded intellectually to varying degrees and to have a number of specific learning difficulties; research also suggests that they are more at risk emotionally and socially than are disabled children without brain disorders [1, 2]. They are, in other words, usually multiply handicapped children. In the UK approximately two-thirds of disabled children thought to need special educational provision are either cerebral-palsied children or children with spina bifida and hydrocephalus, and from what I saw on a brief visit to Canada and the US last October I got the impression that the picture is broadly similar, although I appreciate that the incidence of spina bifida is lower. For this reason I shall talk mainly about disabled children who also have brain dysfunction, in particular about cerebral-palsied and hydrocephalic spina bifida children, since most of my teaching and research experience has been with these groups.

In the main part of this paper I shall try to answer the question: What kinds of physical, intellectual, psychologic, and social problems is the school-age child with a physical disability and accompanying brain dysfunction likely to have?, In the concluding section I shall consider the question: What sort of special educational provision is most appropriate for children with problems such as these?

SPECIAL NEEDS OF THE DISABLED SCHOOLCHILD

Special problems arise for the disabled schoolchild in 3 closely related areas: 1) in physical functioning, 2) in intellectual functioning, and 3) in his emotional and social development. I shall talk very briefly about the first of these and will concentrate on intellectual and social/emotional development.

Physical/Medical Problems

Because the physical problems of disabled children are so obvious they have tended in the UK, at least until fairly recently, to dominate the way in which children are categorized, and this in turn has had a major influence on decisions about where a child goes to school, and to a lesser extent on how his time is spent in school (ie a great emphasis on the therapies). Certainly the child's physical problems will often necessitate changes in the physical environment of the school. These will vary according to the disability but may include modifications to building (ie ramps, lifts, specially designed toilet facilities), modifications to furniture, the provision of special equipment in the classroom, and also the provision of special transport. They are also likely to necessitate special staffing arrangements. Here 2 aspects can be distinguished. First, the child is likely to need personal assistance in coping with physical problems. Help may be needed with toileting, dressing, moving round the school, P.E. and games, supervision of special diets, and so on. Second, and particularly in the case of younger schoolchildren, therapies of different kinds — physiotherapy, speech therapy, occupational therapy — may be required.

In the past it has generally been assumed that these needs could only be met within the framework of a special school; such a placement, however may well be at the expense of the child's social and educational development. Although the situation in the UK is now changing, a substantial minority of disabled children without marked learning disabilities or problems of other kinds are still being placed in the socially and intellectually restricted environment of the special school *primarily* because of their physical or medical needs, for example, because they need intensive physio- or speech therapy, because they are incontinent, or because the local high school has no lift. Disabled children's physical needs *can* be met within ordinary schools, and if we were more resourceful they need never and should never constitute the main reason for placing a child in a restricted social environment.

Special Educational Needs

Next I want to consider briefly the question of intellectual development in disabled children. As I mentioned earlier 2 main groups can be distinguished.

The first comprises children who are motor-handicapped (eg amputees) or otherwise physically disabled (eg children with cystic fibrosis) but have no brain dysfunction. Although the distribution of intelligence in these children is likely to follow a normal pattern, 2 subgroups can be distinguished in terms of actual functioning in school. First, there are those children whose school attainments match their intellectual potential. In my own study of disabled children in ordinary schools [3] I found that generally the motor-handicapped children (most of whom had congenital limb abnormalities) were doing well in reading and almost as well in number work as the nonhandicapped controls.

Second, however, there is some evidence that many disabled children of normal intelligence may be retarded in their attainments. Let me give you 2 examples. In a recent study of children with cystic fibrosis Lindy Burton [4] found that although the mean WISC IQ of the children was 104 and the range of scores well within the limits of normality, 55% of the boys and 66% of the girls were retarded in 2 more basic school subjects to the extent that their test scores were 12 months or more behind those expected of children of their age and intelligence. This was equally true whether the children had been placed in a special school for delicate children or in ordinary schools. The reasons for this retardation are not clear, but children retarded in 2 or more subjects showed a significantly higher level of anxiety on the Taylor Manifest Anxiety Scale than did children retarded in only 1 subject. Burton also suggests that retardation in basic school work may have been fostered by lowered expectations on the part of parents and teachers.

Another example of marked retardation in disabled children of near normal intelligence comes from a study of spina bifida children in South Wales [5] where a very high proportion of those with spina bifida meningocele (mean WISC IQ 93.7) were (despite comparatively mild physical handicaps, an absence of hydrocephalus, and more or less uninterrupted schooling) markedly retarded both in reading and in arithmetic. The reason for the poor attainment level was, to quote the authors, "obscure": however, it seems very likely that in the case of these children and of the children with cystic fibrosis, deprivation of normal experiences in the preschool years may have been one of the major reasons for their later retardation in school.

The other main group of children with developmental disabilities, those with motor disabilities *and* brain dysfunction will generally have some degree of intellectual impairment, with important implications for their education. Most cerebral-palsied children will fall into this category and also most children with spina bifida and hydrocephalus. Since I have just completed research on cognitive functioning in hydrocephalic children [6] let me say a little about this group. Differences between the intellectual functioning of spina bifida children with and without hydrocephalus are marked. The latter, a minority of spina bifida children, appear to be of near normal intelligence, whereas most studies (eg Tew [7] and Spain [8]) show that the mean IQ of hydrocephalic spina bifida children is around 80, with the bulk of the children falling into the 70–90 range. They tend to be, in other words, a borderline group intellectually between normal and mildly mentally retarded children, a fact which has important implications for school placement. There will also be implications for the children's emotional and social development since many will find it a struggle to keep up with their peers. Further difficulties may spring from parental reactions to learning that the child is intellectually impaired. Research with spina bifida children [9] has shown that the parents of children with a mild degree of retardation and apparent good verbal skills have more difficulty in accepting that the child is retarded and may need special provision of some kind than do parents of more severely retarded children, and parental anxiety is very quickly communicated to the child.

Another point with major educational implications is that hydrocephalic children tend, like many cerebral-palsied children, to show an uneven pattern of intellectual functioning. Some aspects of verbal ability (vocabulary skills and the development of syntax) seem normal or near normal, often leading parents, teachers, and others to perceive the children as being brighter than they really are, whereas the children's comprehension and appropriate use of language is often poor. Certain aspects of visual perceptual functioning are usually impaired [10, 11], and figure-ground discrimination is particularly poor [6, 7, 10]. Visuo-motor difficulties are marked and apparent from an early age [8]. While these can be partly accounted for by impaired hand control (arising to a considerable extent from cerebellar damage [6]) the difficulty is by no means one of executing movements only, and there are clear indications that the ability to plan and organize movements in space is impaired. These difficulties affect most school attainments in the basic skills. Many spina bifida children, especially those with IQs below 80 and shunts, are retarded in their reading fluency and even more in reading comprehension; the great majority (probably 4 in 5) have great difficulty in number work and at least 2 in 3 children will have marked difficulties in writing: not only is their writing (like that of many other neurologically impaired children) much slower than that of their peers but it is also poor qualitatively, and this can be a great source of frustration to a child throughout his school life.

Thus many spina bifida children will, like most other disabled children with brain disorders, have marked learning difficulties which may affect the child's concept of himself, his relationship with his peers, the way he is treated by his parents and his teachers, and, most important of all, his school placement.

Emotional and Social Problems

Let me now turn to the emotional, behavioral, and social problems which often occur in disabled school children. These have to be taken into account when decisions about school placement are being made: they may also arise, of course, as a response to a particular type of placement.

There is now quite an extensive literature available on the behavioral and social adjustment of disabled children. This includes, for example, Birch's account [12] of children with minimal brain dysfunction, the studies of Rutter and his colleagues [1, 2] of psychiatric disturbance in disabled children with and without brain disorders, as well as studies of cerebral-palsied children [13, 14] and children with cystic fibrosis [4] to name only a few. Also worth mentioning is the very useful series of annotated bibliographies on the intellectual, social, and emotional development of various groups of disabled children which Doria Pilling of the National Children's Bureau in England has produced [15–18].

A number of general points are raised by these accounts. The first is that children and adults with handicaps that vary greatly in their nature and severity tend to experience the same kinds of emotional, behavioral, and social problems. Whether or not the child is severely or only mildly handicapped appears to be much less crucial than the fact that he may feel "different" from his sibs or his peers and is liable to be treated by them as different when in fact his basic emotional needs, for security and affection, to be accepted by and to be part of a social group, for achievement, recognition and self-expression are identical to theirs. In my own study of disabled children in ordinary schools [3] mildly handicapped children were as likely to be disturbed as those who were severely handicapped and in a recent study of disabled children [2], most of whom were in special schools, the finding was similar. Indeed the authors comment that the severely disabled children "may have been less likely to have psychiatric disorder than those with milder physical impairment," perhaps because those severely disabled find it easier to come to terms with the fact that there are some activities in which they will not be able to participate.

This leads to a second general point: A disabled child's problems are rarely caused directly by the disability (an exception being certain behaviors, such as hyperactivity or distractability, which may be closely associated with organic brain damage), but rather by the reactions of society (including the child's parents, his teachers and his peers) to the disability and also by his own feelings about his disability. Burton [4] in her study of children with cystic fibrosis, (a chronic and possibly life-shortening condition) puts this point very well. "When one considers the development of any chronically sick child, . . . one is assessing behaviour which results not only from the disease but more especially from the whole amalgam of social experiences, hardships, anxieties and evasions which surround it." In particular, however, it seems to be the reactions of the parents to the disability and their way of coping which has by far the greatest influence on the child's adjustment. If they worry about it, so does he. If they are ashamed, he will be sensitive too. If they regard it objectively, he is more likely to be able to accept it as a fact. Unfortunately parents of handicapped children still tend to have few opportunities of discussing their feelings about the handicap and the way in which this affects their management of the child.

A third point suggested by research is that although children disabled in different ways tend to have the same kinds of problems, those who have brain disorders in addition to motor impairment are more at risk of becoming emotionally and behaviorally disturbed. In the epidemiologic study carried out by Rutter and his colleagues [1] in the Isle of Wight among 10–11-year-olds, the rate of psychiatric disorder was more than twice as high (24%) in "neurologically abnormal" children (this group included mainly cerebral-palsied, spina bifida, and epileptic children) as it was in children with "physical disorders" (eg asthma or heart disease) and no neurologic abnormalities (9%), and they in turn showed a higher rate of disorders than the general 10–11-year-old population (6%).

Since the children with brain disorders differed markedly from those with physical disorders in that they were of lower intelligence and also more obviously disabled, a further study was set up in which these factors were better controlled [2]. In this study children with brain disorders and a mean IQ of 90.7 (all had either cerebral palsy or hydrocephalus) were compared with children with a variety of physical disorders (including polio, muscular dystrophy, and skeletal defects or deformities) but no upper brain stem damage (mean IQ 100.8). An overall assessment of psychiatric disorder was made on the basis of teacher and parent questionnaires and interviews with the parents, teachers, and child, and it was found that 24% of the brain-lesion group showed a psychiatric disorder with substantial social impairment, compared with only 12% of the other group. The authors conclude that "it is highly probable that the brain damage as such was responsible for the children's increased vulnerability to emotional and behavioural problems." However, they also emphasize that three-quarters of the brain-damaged children did not have psychiatric problems, and even among the children who did the problems varied in type, ie there was no stereotyped behavioral picture. As in the case of nonhandicapped children and of disabled children without brain damage, disturbed behavior was much more common in children from overcrowded homes, broken homes, families with marital discord, or homes where the mother had psychiatric problems. Children with low IQs and/or reading retardation were also somewhat more at risk psychiatrically.

PARTICULAR PROBLEMS

Having made those rather general points I would like to talk in a little more detail about 3 kinds of problems which are very commonly encountered in schoolchildren with developmental disabilities and brain disorders. These are 1) the problem of distractability; 2) fearful, anxious, and unsociable behavior, and 3) the effects of developmental disabilities upon social maturity and peer relationships. My selection of these topics may seem rather arbitrary to you, but in the short time available I have had to be selective, and I think that these are all important issues.

Distractability

Most accounts of research with hydrocephalic and with cerebral-palsied children as well as reports from teachers suggest that distractability is a major problem. In their South Wales study of spina bifida children, Tew and Laurence [19] asked teachers to estimate the length of time the child was usually able to concentrate on basic school subjects: the average time reported for the controls was 18 min, for the children with shunt-controlled hydrocephalus only 9 min. In my own study [3] of disabled children in ordinary primary schools, 88% of the children with cerebral palsy or hydrocephalus were rated by teachers as having poor concentration, compared with only 43% of the disabled children without neurologic involvement and 36% of the nonhandicapped children, respectively. Distractable children tend to react continuously to inessential stimuli which may be visual, auditory, or tactile and may also have difficulty in focusing attention and in maintaining it on the relevant stimulus.

Many researchers have suggested a causal link between attentional problems and neurologic impairment; one commonly held theory is that the neurologic impairment is such that the child has not the normal ability to filter out or inhibit irrelevant incoming stimuli. In this respect children with neurologic abnormalities may function like younger normal children who tend, as Turnure [20] has shown, to be quite easily distracted by irrelevant cues up to the age of about 6.5–7.5 years.

However, attentional problems cannot be assumed to result from neurologic abnormalities alone, and other factors must be taken into account. A child with spina bifida for example, may from quite an early age, have been given toys which were unsuited to his level of functioning, perhaps because of difficulties in manipulation or perception. Activities that are too demanding do not usually hold a child's attention for long and the result may be that the child fails to develop the ability to concentrate. Research on the attention span of young normal children is interesting in this context. Moyer and Gilmer [21, 22] have shown that age is much less important than the stimulus material and its "drawing power" and that even children as young as 18 months can concentrate for relatively long periods of time (up to half an hour) with one toy if they have the right toy. The relationship between the nature of the task and the presence or absence of distractable behavior has also been explored by Sen [23]. Her subjects were young, mentally retarded adults, and she found that although they were more likely to show distractable behavior than normal adults, distractors (eg background noise) had comparatively little effect when the level of the task was well suited to the subject's capabilities. Task difficulty may thus contribute to distractability in spina bifida and other disabled children.

Social factors may also play a part. Disabled children often depend heavily in the early years upon adults, both at home and in hospital, to meet their physical needs. It becomes important for the child to pay attention to the visual and verbal cues given out by adults and for him to develop ways of gaining their attention. Children may become more sensitized to social stimuli than to the stimuli present in the toy or the book and so may never actually learn to pay attention for long to any one activity. Adults may inadvertently reinforce inattentive and inappropriate behavior by smiling or cuddling or praise and fail to reward the child for actually concentrating on a task.

Whatever the reasons for the distractable behavior which characterizes many disabled children with brain disorders, it undoubtedly adds to the child's problems both in the preschool period, when the child often does not concentrate on any one activity for long enough to benefit from it, and, more obviously, at school. Parents, teachers, and others working with children with brain lesions should therefore be alerted to the existence of this problem and be taught how to tackle it, and here I think behavior-modification techniques have a great deal to offer.

Fears and Anxieties

Rutter [24] and his colleagues have divided childhood psychiatric disorders into the 3 subtypes: 1) predominantly antisocial or conduct disorders (ie abnormal behavior which gives rise to social disapproval); 2) neurotic disorders (ie an abnormality of the emotions such as disproportionate anxiety); and 3) the mixed type. In general, research with disabled children suggests that neurotic or emotional disorders are more common in disabled children than conduct disorders, especially in children with brain lesions [2, 3]. In hydrocephalic spina bifida children, for example, the absence of antisocial behavior is quite marked and is replaced by "good" but unsociable and often rather passive behavior [25]. The comments of an organizer of playgroups for spina bifida children are interesting [26]: "Restricted mobility means that the child cannot release his feelings, by running, jumping or other energetic movements. Long periods in hospital and the anxious care of adults on whom he must depend also control his freedom in this respect. In his attempts to deal with his experiences he generally learns to inhibit emotions he considers dangerous or painful, particularly anger ... and so becomes passive, apathetic, obedient and 'good'." "Good" but "unsociable" behavior of a similar kind, where the child is afraid of new tasks and new situations and timid with people, has also been commented on by Burton [4, pp. 172–3] in children with cystic fibrosis.

The fearfulness and anxiety often seen in disabled children with brain disorders can take several forms. A fear of failure is common, and the child may refuse to attempt a new task or require much encouragement and constant reassurance that he is doing all right. Apprehension about new situations is also noticeable: a spina bifida child, for example, may refuse to go on an expedition with the rest of his class. One reason for this is that he may not know how he will cope physically, and it often helps to spend considerable time describing in advance (as one might to a younger child) the sequence of events, including the arrangements for toileting and so on. Burton [4, 27] has observed similar reactions in children with asthma and with cystic fibrosis and comments that "sick children seem to develop a special and understandable defensiveness in order to ward off occurrences which might prove stressful for them."

Anxieties about peer reactions to handicaps, including "invisible" aspects of the handicap, are also common. Incontinence, a major handicap for most spina bifida children, provides a good example. It might be expected that those children whose incontinence has been reasonably reliably controlled by the wearing of a urinary appliance or by a urinary diversion (referred to hereafter as "continent" children) would have fewer emotional and social problems than those who were often uncontrollably wet or soiled ("incontinent" children), but the small amount of evidence we have so far suggests that this is not necessarily so, and also that boys and girls may react differently to having to depend on urinary appliances. Fulthorpe [28] in a study of 12 incontinent and 21 continent spina bifida children attending a residential school for physically handicapped children found no significant overall differences in the Bristol Social Adjustment Guide scores of the incontinent and continent children. However, the findings differed considerably according to the sex of the child. The boys who had been made continent by the fitting of a urinary appliance tended to show unsociable social behavior, (lack of self-assertion, apprehension about new situations and tasks, withdrawal, and lack of initiative), while it was the incontinent boys who were more forthcoming. Fulthorpe suggests that the wearing of a penile bag may emphasize feelings of being different and become an increasingly acute problem as the boy grows older. This was also a finding in a study of teenagers with spina bifida carried out by Steven Dorner of Great Ormond Street Hospital [29]. The social isolation of many of these teenagers was marked, and although isolation and impaired mobility were closely associated, boys who were mobile often stayed at home because of anxieties connected with the wearing of urinary appliances.

In contrast to the boys, the girls who had had urinary diversions were significantly better adjusted than the incontinent girls, who showed marked symptoms of anxiety, inferiority, and inadequacy and were easily disheartened and upset. Fulthorpe suggests that the girls may have been more aware than the boys of the social problems likely to arise from their incontinence and that these realizations may have fostered "feelings of inadequacy and apprehensiveness."

On the whole the little evidence we have suggests that while incontinence may give rise to emotional problems it is not a major social problem in school. The incontinent spina bifida children in my study [3] of disabled children in ordinary schools were chosen as friends as often as continent disabled children who had no such problems; the only children in this study who were teased because they were "smelly" were 2 enuretic control group children who came from very deprived homes. However, teachers and other adults should realize that almost all spina bifida children, in whatever kind of school, are deeply ashamed of their incontinence and worried in case their peers discover that they wear special appliances. Staff can help, first by ensuring that the children have toileting privacy, and second by making sure that the child knows there is a named adult who has been informed about his problem and to whom he can go for help. It is also helpful for the teacher and parents to discuss the handling of this problem (eg what the other children are going to be told) before the incontinent child joins the class.

Anxiety connected with incontinence is only one example of the many anxieties disabled children may have about their handicaps. Because many disabled children "cause no trouble" in school, adults often wrongly assume an absence of emotional stress when the child probably has anxieties which it would be helpful for him to be able to discuss. Burton's experience [4] with children with cystic fibrosis is relevant here. She found that the parents, burdened with the problems of the day-to-day physical care of the child, had little energy left for worrying about his emotional feelings concerning his handicap. As a result only 32% of the school-age children in her study had felt able to talk over their illness with anyone. When the subject was sympathetically broached by the interviewer they were glad to speak of their feelings, and 65% expressed a fear of being hurt, 50% of being ill, and 47% of going into hospital, while 58% said the illness made them sad and 36% said it worried them. There is of course a crucial difference between children with cystic fibrosis and many other disabling conditions insofar as the former are much more likely to become seriously ill. However, growing appreciation of physical limitations, increasing self-consciousness about being "different," and apprehension about the future are anxieties shared by most disabled children.

Social Problems

Let me turn next to look very briefly at some of the social implications of severe disability. There are 2 closely related aspects of this which I want to discuss in relation to children of primary school age. The first is the question of social maturity and the second of peer relationships.

Social maturity. Many disabled children are much less independent socially than are their peers, and this will inevitably affect peer relationships. In part lack of social maturity springs directly from the physical limitations imposed by the child's handicap. Also important is the fact that many disabled children are treated by parents, sibs, or other adults as younger than they really are and are given insufficient encouragement in developing social independence.

Social maturity is something which is difficult to measure, particularly in the case of disabled children, since the main scales used for this purpose (the Vineland Scale of Social Maturity [30] and the Manchester Scales of Social Adaptation [31]) contain many items which depend on a child's physical status (eg ability to dress himself, go to the shops alone or to the park). Since these will be impossible for a severely handicapped child his scores may be somewhat misleading in that socially he might be more mature (for example, in terms of making decisions for himself) than his low scores would suggest.

However, most studies do indicate a very marked retardation in social skills in disabled children [3, 7, 28]. In my own study of disabled children in ordinary schools [3] in which I used the Manchester Scales of Social Adaptation I found, predictably, that on the "self-direction" scales, covering socialization of play, freedom of movement, self help, handling of money and responsibility in the home, there was a clear gradation in performance depending on severity of handicap, with the mildly handicapped children making the highest scores and the severely handicapped the lowest. However, less expected was the fact that the children with brain dysfunction showed significantly lower levels of social competence in all these areas than the disabled children without brain dysfunction although the 2 groups were very similar in terms of the severity of their handicaps. Some of the differences were most striking and suggested that parents of cerebral-palsied and hydrocephalic children may have been over-solicitous: for example, only 4% of the brain dysfunction group went to school unaccompanied, compared with 75% of the other disabled children and 90% of the controls. The same differences occurred inside the home: only 15% of this group helped with simple household chores, compared with 56% of the other disabled children and 63% of the controls.

Peer relationships. I shall only say a little about this subject since it has already been discussed extensively by Professor Richardson (this volume). The extent to which a disabled child is accepted by his peers seems to depend more on personality factors and also on intellectual level than on the severity of the physical handicap. My own study of disabled children placed individually in ordinary schools suggested that the amount and quality of social integration both inside and outside school was very encouraging, and one of the conclusions I reached was that social problems were, at least for children of this age group, much less marked than intellectual problems.

This is not to say that social problems are totally absent. The result of sociometric testing in my study showed that the disabled children were chosen less often as friends than the controls. Severity of handicap did not appear to affect the child's social acceptability, indeed, as I mentioned earlier in connection with emotional disturbance, the mildly handicapped children seemed slightly more at risk of social isolation than those who were severely handicapped. It was also the case that the children with brain disorders seemed more at risk of being isolated (15% received no friendship choices) than disabled children without brain disorders (only 6% of this group being isolated, compared with 3% of the controls). Within the brain disorder group cerebral-palsied children seemed less well accepted than those with spina bifida and hydrocephalus, particularly if they were boys.

The numbers in my study were too small to provide more than clues about which disabled children may be most vulnerable socially: further research is needed into whether and if so why cerebral-palsied children tend to have more difficulty than other disabled children in peer relationships, and also, as I indicated earlier, to be less independent socially. Are parents of cerebral-palsied children in fact more protective than parents of other disabled children? How important a factor is intellectual retardation? Do the child's appearance and/or speech make it more difficult for his peers to accept him than, for example, a child with spina bifida and hydrocephalus and obvious lower-limb paralysis? Are cerebral-palsied children who have been integrated from the preschool level on better accepted than those who join regular classes at an older age? How far can explanations on the part of the teacher help?

I have not mentioned teasing: this I found to be only a minor problem for disabled children in ordinary schools, particularly if the child had attended an ordinary school from an early age. It was mainly confined to name-calling and although parent reports indicated more teasing to be going on than teachers were aware of, this is a problem with which children and teachers are generally able to cope. What we should be equally concerned about is the disabled child, often cerebral-palsied and often only mildly handicapped, who causes no trouble to the teachers and may not even be noticed but has no real friends in school. There is also the problem of the opposite kind, that some disabled children have far too much done for them by over-helpful peers. It is not always enough to encourage the disabled child to do all he can for himself: it may also be necessary to explain to his peers what he can do or is learning to do for himself and why it is important that he is allowed to, and here the teacher's own behavior will provide an important model for the class.

A final point which needs to be made about peer relationships is that teachers and other adults tend to be more concerned about the social behavior of non-handicapped children than about that of the disabled child. The former should not be expected to make allowances all the time for demanding, or socially inappropriate, or unattractive behavior in a disabled child. He too has to learn certain social skills and must be helped by his teachers to modify behavior which the other children may correctly perceive as assertive, self-centered, withdrawn, or babyish. Disabled children most in need of such help in developing social skills are generally those who have spent much of their time in special classes or special schools. They often have very little opportunity to develop normal social skills outside the classroom since at home, particularly in the holidays, they are frequently lonely and isolated.

SPECIAL EDUCATIONAL PROVISION FOR DISABLED CHILDREN

Let me now turn to the concluding part of my paper. Here my main question is, what sort of school environment will be most appropriate for a child with the kinds of physical, intellectual, and perhaps also social and behavioral problems which I have outlined so far? Clearly a large proportion of children with developmental disabilities will, because of their physical or emotional or intellectual problems, or a combination of these, need special education. For many people, certainly in the UK, special education still means special schools. A more useful approach which has been adopted by the Council for Exceptional Children here [32] is to think in terms of a *continuum* of provision, ranging from placement of a child in an ordinary class with no modifications to placement in highly specialized residential institutions. The main points along the continuum are: 1) ordinary class full-time with no extra help; 2) ordinary class full-time but ancillary help provided; 3) ordinary class (child's base) part-time but withdrawn part-time to "resource room" or similar special facility; 4) special class (base) part-time, ordinary class for selected activities only; 5) special class full-time other than for social activities (meals, playtime, etc); 6) day special school (base) formally linked to an ordinary school; 7) day special school without such links; 8) boarding special school; 9) residential hospital school.

The situation in the UK at present is that disabled children tend either to be placed in ordinary classes without extra help or in day or residential special schools. Comparatively few are in the types of placement suggested in nos. 2–5, that is, receiving special schooling within ordinary schools in which supportive services have been provided, although I believe that here in the US this type of provision is now being widely developed.

Let me say a few words about the different ways of organizing special provision in ordinary schools. In type 2 provision the child is in an ordinary class but special supportive services are available to him and/or his teacher. What these are depend on the nature of the handicap. Physically handicapped children may be provided with a personal assistant whose activities could include supervision and help with toileting, dressing, feeding, or mobility. In some areas physiotherapy, speech therapy, and occupational therapy is provided by mobile teams. In addition teachers may be supported by peripatetic specialists whose duties may be largely advisory or may include individual teaching.

Type 3 provision (in an ordinary class but supported by a school resource center) is now being very widely used in Sweden, where it is national policy to place *all* handicapped children in ordinary schools [33, 34], to a lesser extent in

Denmark, and also, I understand, in parts of the US [32, 35]. In Sweden, the resource room coupled with the extensive use of companion teachers who work with the child in the regular classroom is fast replacing special classes (which in their turn have replaced most special schools) as the main way in which special education is provided. Resource centers can be established in selected schools for children with a variety of handicaps, including slow learners, physically handicapped children with additional learning difficulties, hearing or visually impaired children, and disturbed children, the child being withdrawn to the specially staffed and specially equipped resource center for as much individual help as he requires.

The other main way of organizing special schooling within the ordinary school is the special class (types 4 and 5). The aim is generally to cut down, gradually, the time the child spends there and to increase his participation not only in the social but also the intellectual activities of the rest of the school. However, for some children, for example, severely retarded children, social integration may be the only meaningful form of integration to aim at and the child's base may always be the special class. In Britain special classes have been widely used for mildly retarded children but less often for other groups. In Sweden, although still widely used for severely retarded children, special classes are being replaced by resource centers, partly because, as is frequently pointed out [36], children in special classes can be very isolated.

Certainly the trends in Scandinavia, in North America, and to a much more limited extent, in the UK to develop special educational services within ordinary schools are very much to be welcomed. Provision of the kinds I have outlined has the potential for giving disabled children (and their teachers) the very specialized help and support they need intellectually and emotionally, while at the same time maximizing their opportunities for interacting socially with their nonhandicapped peers. However, surprisingly little evaluation of the effectiveness of different ways of providing these children with special services has been done, and we still need more hard research evidence of 2 main kinds. First, we need to know more about the best way of organizing services for disabled children. Is the regular class coupled with a resource room in a physically adapted school, the model toward which we should be aiming for *most* disabled children? Which children, if any, will it not be suitable for? Do we need different models for children of different ages? Second, even if this way of organizing services is found to be feasible, we still have only a framework. What matters ultimately is what can be done to improve the quality of the learning and social experiences which take place within that framework.

REFERENCES

1. Rutter, M., Tizard, J., and Whitmore, J. (eds.): "Education, Health and Behaviour." London: Longmans, 1970.

2. Seidel, U. P., Chadwick, O. F. D., and Rutter, M.: Psychological disorders in crippled children. A comparative study of children with and without brain damage. Dev. Med. Child. Neurol. 17:563–573, 1975.
3. Anderson, E. M.: "The Disabled Schoolchild: A Study of Integration in Primary Schools." London: Methuen & Co., New York: Barnes and Noble, 1973.
4. Burton, L.: "The Family Life of Sick Children." London: Routledge and Kegan Paul, 1975.
5. Tew, B. J., and Laurence, K. M.: The ability and attainments of spina bifida patients born in S. Wales between 1956–62. Dev. Med. Child. Neurol. (Suppl.) 27:124–131, 1972.
6. Anderson, E. M.: Cognitive and motor deficits in children with spina bifida and hydrocephalus with special reference to writing difficulties. (Ph.D. Thesis, University of London.)
7. Tew, B. J.: Spina bifida and hydrocephalus: Facts, fallacies and future. Spec. Educ. 62(4): 26–31, 1973.
8. Spain, B.: Verbal and performance ability in pre-school children with spina bifida. Dev. Med. Child. Neurol. 16:773–780, 1974.
9. Tew, B. J., Payne, H., Laurence, K. M., and Rawnsley, K.: Psychological testing: Reactions of parents of physically handicapped and normal children. Dev. Med. Child. Neurol. 16(4):501–506, 1974.
10. Dodds, J.: Hydrocephalic children and visual perception. (M. Ed. Psychol. Master's Dissertation, University of Sussex.)
11. Ball, M.: Investigation into the reading abilities and related perceptual abilities of spina bifida children. (Submitted for Master's degree in Child Development, University of London.)
12. Birch, H. G.: "Brain Damage in Children." Baltimore: Williams and Wilkins, 1964.
13. Nielsen, H. H.: "A Psychological Study of Cerebral-palsied Children." Copenhagen: Munksgaard, 1966.
14. Oswin, M.: "Behaviour Problems Among Children With Cerebral Palsy." Bristol: John Wright and Sons, 1967.
15. Pilling, D.: The orthopaedically handicapped child. Social, emotional and educational adjustment: An annotated bibliography. Windsor, Berks: NFER, 1972.
16. Pilling, D.: The child with cerebral palsy. An annotated bibliography. Windsor, Berks.: NFER, 1973a.
17. Pilling, D.: The child with spina bifida. An annotated bibliography. Windsor, Berks.: NFER, 1973b.
18. Pilling, D.: The child with a chronic medical problem. An annotated bibliography. Windsor, Berks.: NFER, 1974.
19. Tew, B. J., and Laurence, K. M.: The effects of hydrocephalus on intelligence, visual perception and school attainment. Dev. Med. Child. Neurol. (Suppl.) 35:129–134, 1975.
20. Turnure, J. E.: Children's reactions to distractors in a learning situation. Dev. Psychol. 2(1):115–122, 1970.
21. Moyer, K. E., and Gilmer, B. V. H.: The concept of attention spans in children. Elementary School Journal 54:464–466, 1954.
22. Moyer, K. E., and Gilmer, B. V. H.: Attention spans of children for experimentally designed toys. J. Genet. Psychol. 87:187–201, 1955.
23. Sen, A.: Factors affecting distractability in the subnormal: An experimental investigation. (Ph.D. Dissertation, University of Hull.)
24. Rutter, M.: A children's behaviour questionnaire for completion by teachers: Preliminary findings. J. Child Psychol. Psychiatry 8:1–11, 1967.

25. Anderson, E. M., and Spain. B.: "The Child With Spina Bifida." London: Methuen & Co. (In press.)
26. Hodges, D. E. S.: Handicapped adventure. In Boswell, D. M. and Wingrove, J. M. (eds.): "The Handicapped Person in the Community." London: Tavistock, 1974.
27. Burton, L.: "Vulnerable Children." London: Routledge and Kegan Paul, 1968.
28. Fulthorpe, D.: Spina bifida: Some psychological aspects. Spec. Ed. 1 (4): 17–20, 1974.
29. Dorner, S.: Adolescents with spina bifida – how they see their situation. Arch. Dis. Child. (In press.)
30. Doll, E. A.: "The Vineland Social Maturity Scale." Minneapolis, Minn.: Educational Test Bureau, 1947.
31. Lunzer, E. A.: "Manchester Scales of Social Adaptation." Windsor, Berks.: NFER, 1966.
32. Educational Facilities Laboratory: One out of ten – school planning for the handicapped. EFL Special Education Project, 477 Madison Avenue, New York, N.Y. 10022, 1974.
33. Lundstrom, K.: Open special education, how to initiate, develop and follow up a programme of integrated education. Paper read at 5th International Seminar on Special Education, Melbourne, 1972.
34. Stenholm, B.: The teaching of children with educational difficulties and handicaps in Sweden. Stockholm: Swedish Institute, 1975.
35. Birch, J. W.: "Mainstreaming: Educable Mentally Retarded Children in Regular Classes." Minneapolis, Minn.: Publ. Leadership Training Institute/Special Education, University of Minnesota, 1974,
36. Department of Education and Science: Integrating handicapped children. D. E. S. Information Section, London, 1974.

Adolescence — A Period of Stress, the Search for an Identity

Thomas E. Strax, MD

The development of the child appears as a succession of periods. Each of these extends the preceding period, reconstructs it on a new level, and then later surpasses it. Occasionally, there is an arrest of the maturation process. This is much more common in the disabled individual, and will be discussed in this paper. I intend to talk about this problem in terms of adolescence. I will draw upon information derived from the literature and from personal and clinical experience.

Adolescence is a period of "storm and stress" characterized by biologic, social, and emotional changes. The adolescent must consolidate his identity, achieve independence from his parents, establish new love objects outside the family, and find a vocation. The actual time period varies from culture to culture and is modified by socioeconomic factors within a culture. Among the poor, this can be an extremely short period of time, with the adolescent becoming independent between ages 15 to 18. In the middle class, adolescence might extend through college, even graduate school, with the individual still being controlled by the family mantle and being supported by it [1].

Achieving the 4 major developmental tasks during a period of biologic stress is extremely difficult for the normal individual. These tasks are made even more difficult with a physical disability. This paper will limit itself to physically disabled children with intact families and average intelligence.

The disabled individual almost always has a prolonged adolescence for several reasons: 1) he has been overprotected and sheltered; 2) most of his growth must come from his nuclear and extended family, because his experiences with peers are limited. The identity crisis is even more profound because of a dearth of appropriate role models [2–5].

Maturation and the achievement of adolescent goals do not occur smoothly but progress in a jerky, chaotic fashion. This causes stress. The intent of this paper is to discuss the various forms of adolescent stress, the manner in which it is handled, and the special problems encountered by the physically disabled [1, 6, 7].

The stresses encountered in achieving the goals of adolescence can be expressed in many different ways: for example, new hairstyles, new forms of dress, hero worship, working hard at school, or being very active in sports. Other ways of handling stress, such as rebellion against one's parents, can be accomplished by an acting out peer group. Acting out might take the form of truancy, delinquency, sexual abuse, and drug addiction [6, 7]. Many of these outlets are not available to the disabled.

In order to deal with the painful realities of rejection, scorn, and/or embarrassment, the disabled adolescent might (occasionally) resort to such devices as fantasy and denial. Depending on their intensity and frequency, these defense mechanisms need not be pathologic.

Despite the extensive literature on the psychologic problems of adolescence, there is a dearth of information on the predicament of the physically disabled teenager [8, 9].

To find one's identity, one must first have an intact image of one's own body, be able to fantasize different identities, and see how those roles fit. The first identity figures are parents. As the adolescent enlarges his or her horizon, the choice of identities goes beyond the family to rock figures, presidents, lawyers, doctors, and so on. The number of figures available depends upon culture, economic status, and experience. The disabled child in the wheelchair does not often get a chance to go to baseball games or wander around downtown. The disabled adolescent is also limited as to the number of individuals he can fantasize being and still relate to reality. Somebody in a wheelchair cannot be a baseball player.

How we see ourselves in relationship to the perceived ideal of our society is extremely important. Most of this is controlled by predisposing attitudes. Friedman [2], in his doctoral dissertation, reviews a study by Sandbourne in 1966 where 62 disabled children and 361 nondisabled children from 14 elementary school classes were tested. Each child was given 3 criteria to choose from: playmates, friends, and workmates. Physically handicapped children were chosen significantly fewer times, and those with orthopedic handicaps were chosen last.

Centers and Centers [10] in 1963 found that amputee children were often rejected by their normal peers. They felt that the presence of an amputation represented a threat to body integrity. Tringo [11] in 1970 investigated the attitudes of nondisabled high school, college undergraduate and graduate students, and rehabilitation workers toward 21 specific disabilities. He found that subjects with higher educational levels showed less rejection of disabled persons. There were 9 possible ratings from which to choose. The range varied from: "would marry" to "would put to death." Increased education levels seem to decrease social distance scores. The highest ranking brain-injured type was epilepsy, which ranked 13 out of 22. Familiarity and experience with specific disabilities may have been responsible for the ratings assigned them. Cancer, stroke, and heart disease are common in all families and thus had a high rating. Alcoholism and criminal experiences tended to have a low position in the study. Yuker et al [12] in 1970 found that close personal contact with a disabled person resulted in greater acceptance of a particular disability. Persons having disabled family members and professionals working with the disabled had little change in their attitudes with increased contact. It was felt that a rehabilitation setting provided information which stressed the limitations of the disabled. Friedman [2] studied the effects of modeling on choosing acceptable playmates among nondisabled children, disabled children in wheelchairs, and facially disfigured children. His models represented the highest, the middle, and the low preferential groups. He used children from the 7th to the 12th grades. Nondisabled children, wheelchair-bound children, and facially disfigured children all modeled identically. They chose as friends nondisabled first, wheelchair-bound second, and facially disfigured third.

Self-acceptance must come before anybody else can accept a disabled individual. These studies demonstrate a reluctance of the physically normal child to accept the physically disabled child into his peer group. Therefore, the disabled adolescent is deprived of a valuable tool in working out his adolescent problems. The ostracizing of the disabled by the normal adolescent appears to be based, in part, on lack of experience with the disabled and their fear of becoming disabled. By the time a physically disabled child becomes an adolescent he or she is aware of society's ideal physical image. Like his normal peers, he will also reject a physically disabled adolescent and will also reject himself. An individual's self-image is usually based upon society's norm [7, 13, 14]. We look better and are more perfect in our dreams. Nobody is satisfied with the way his voice sounds on a tape recorder or the way he looks in a mirror. It is my personal and professional experience that paraplegics and other disabled persons with marked gait problems see themselves in their dreams as walking normally (most of the time).

It is very difficult to deny one's physical disability when one walks toward a reflecting surface or enters a crowd of people with similar disabilities. The most anxiety-producing summer that I ever had was that between my second and third year in medical school. I had been offered and had accepted a summer fellowship to work with disabled children. Most of these children had cerebral palsy, and because of my own disability I was forced to face things about myself which I had rejected or had denied.

Independence from parents has 2 elements. One is emotional independence, and the other is financial independence. The disabled child is usually babied (infantilized) more than the able-bodied child and, therefore, is much more dependent on the parent. He is afraid of loss of parental love and of eventual loss of parent. Parents who encourage a certain amount of independence in normal adolescents, often overprotect their physically disabled adolescent [3, 6].

The child who has been overprotected grows into an individual who feels that he may need special protection. This, coupled with the special needs of the physically disabled, creates an infantile and immature personality. The disabled child has been treated differently. He or she has not had to live up to the same rules and regulations that control the lives of other family members.

The adolescent is constantly struggling with his parents. He openly rejects and criticizes their viewpoints. At times, he is angry when his parents fail to set limits, but on other occasions he vehemently opposes any delineation of privileges [6, 7, 15].

The adolescent is constantly seeking to find flaws in his parents' behavior and personality. He looks for reasons to criticize or doubt their judgment. The arguments which ensue instill a feeling of guilt and hostility in both the parent and child. In the case of the physically disabled adolescent, separation from parents is extremely difficult. This is due to decreased mobility, which might be real as in the case of a child in a wheelchair or wearing braces and crutches, or may be psychologic in the case of the parent who forbids his physically disabled youngster from going out with his peer group to ball games or to see movies [3, 6, 7, 15].

When they finally enter the outside world, schools segregate such youths into special classes. Peer groups will not admit them; without friends they find life extremely lonely. In an attempt to find friends and attract attention, the disabled are more prone to turn toward inappropriate behavior such as loud talking and behaving foolishly. The normal adolescent who turns to this type of behavior usually gets instant feedback from family, teachers, and peer group members. This is not so with the physically disabled who is usually pitied and coddled.

Children who are considered disabled by their parents and have not been admitted to peer groups have a great deal of difficulty when they get to school. They feel that they are inferior. They usually need some special attention because of incoordination, writing, and speaking problems. Many of the children with physical disabilities have learning problems due to emotional disorders. They fail to meet their parents' expectations. This, coupled with their inability to be accepted within a peer group, leads to complete withdrawal. In junior and senior high school there is generally a need for greater mobility. Physical and learning disabilities may be aggravated by entry into adolescence [7, 15, 16].

Many of the parents I see are afraid to allow their children to be integrated into society. They feel that their child can only be hurt. The normal parent expects the child to eventually leave home. This is not so of the parent with the physically disabled child. This child is forever a child and is forever protected. I was extremely lucky. My parents felt that the most important thing they could give me was the ability to exist in society on my own two feet. To do this, I had to be integrated into society. When the Cub Scouts wouldn't take me, my mother started her own pack for the children in the neighborhood. When the schools wouldn't accept me, they went to court. When the bus driver wouldn't let me ride, they forced him to through the president of the affiliated union.

Parents should, if possible, encourage their disabled child to grow and be treated as any other child. It is important for the emotional maturation of the child to be accepted into a neighborhood peer group.

The next question is what do we do with the severely physically involved individual who cannot move around a school situation and, therefore, needs a special class and a special school. This child must also be integrated into society if he or she is to live a life within that society.

Segregation versus integration of the disabled is a difficult problem. Neither special schools nor isolated environments are being advocated in this paper. There have been studies to show that the disabled child can learn better when he is with a homogeneous peer group, instead of in a 40-pupil class which is moving at a rate that he or she cannot handle. The only problem with this type of isolation is that at some point the individual must be integrated into society. This is difficult if integration has not been occurring all along.

At the onset of puberty, a child's life is centered in the family, but it is shortly transferred to an influential peer group. Intense friendships are made first with members of the same sex and later in adolescence with members of the opposite sex. Family-centered orientation diminishes and peer values become more important. If the adolescent does not find or is not admitted to a peer group, serious difficulties will develop [1, 6, 7]. Assimilation into a peer group provides the adolescent with a vehicle for separation from the home. The earlier the entry into a peer group the quicker the emotional milestones needed for independence will be passed. The normal child has outside friends when he starts to walk, between 1 and 3 years. Lessons learned during this early playing are needed for later maturation. By 5 or 6 the normal child is ready for school and knows how to make friends and play with other children. The physically disabled child may not be walking until 5 or 6 and is, therefore, denied the outside influence of a peer group. By the time adolescence comes around, this child is far behind the emotional maturation of the physically normal child and lacks the experience of how to handle peer relationships and later on, social and sexual relationships.

Some physically disabled children have poor coordination. They have difficulty in dressing, holding a pencil, and find it difficult to keep up with their peer group in the areas of athletics and scholastics. It is agonizing for a physically disabled or uncoordinated youngster, who has trouble dancing, conversing, or participating in sports activities, to join in with other teenagers.

Williams [17] in 1970 discussed alienation syndrome in adolescence. He pointed out that our society reinforces narcissistic competitive individualism with emphasis on performance, achievement, and productivity at the expense of relationships both in the family and with peer groups. As a result, one cannot establish a successful relationship later on in adolescence and in adult life.

A fast moving, achievement-oriented society does not have a place for a slow individual. It is not fashionable to have disabled friends or to slow down for someone who needs some help. During my middle teens, I found that many of my friends would leave me home when they went to ball games or when out on the town. The only outlet for my depression was studying.

Dorner [18] and his study of *spina bifida* youngsters found that the non-handicapped friends of preadolescence were lost during adolescence. About half of his adolescents were judged to be severely socially isolated. In his group the more mobile the *spina bifida* adolescent was, the less the social isolation. Depression was extremely common. Of the girls and boys studied, 31% and 15%, respectively, had persistent periods of depression or suicidal ideas. Anxiety about the future was extremely common, primarily over employment, independence from family, and the possibility of marriage

The function of late adolescence is to establish new objects outside of the family and a vocational goal. These functions cannot really be undertaken until the adolescent has been able to accomplish 1) consolidating an identity for him- or herself, and 2) achieving a semblance of independence from the family and acceptance into a peer group.

The disabled adolescent enters late adolescence socially deprived and immature. He does not know how to approach or handle himself with somebody of the same sex let alone someone of the opposite sex. The social aspect of school and peer group activities has usually been absent.

To the above problems we have to add that we are dealing with: 1) an indivual who is an outcast, not acceptable to society; and 2) the individual who is usually full of self-pity and egocentricity.

The physically disabled have also rejected themselves. Subconsciously, they worry and wonder if their defective bodies will function. The physically disabled are less mobile and, therefore, have less chance of meeting appropriate mates and being able to court in the usual fashion available to his peer group [3, 7, 10, 11]. If the disabled person has developed the emotional maturity, self-esteem, and confidence needed to find a mate, he must now deal with the problem of not being acceptable to people of the opposite sex.

Vocational aspirations usually have similar problems as the above, and I will not go into the special problems in this particular paper.

I remember adolescence as being extremely painful. My close childhood friends down the block rejected me during adolescence and went off with other friends who were able to date, play ball, and run around. Most of my time was spent either in fantasy or by compensation through school achievement. I would spend hours listening to rock and roll music and feeling sorry for myself. It was not until I entered college during late adolescence that I was able to shake my depression by finding an accepting peer group.

It is extremely important for any adolescent, disabled included, that he or she not be coddled but instead be accepted on the same basis as any other member of the peer group. If the disabled youth is treated specially, he will continue to remain dependent and retain the image of a second class citizen. I was extremely lucky in this respect in that I found a group that would not tolerate self-pity. This assisted me in developing the toughness essential to function in a heterogeneous, often ambiguously changing society.

In summary, for the disabled, adolescence is a period of self-examination and rejection. Hopefully, it will be followed by a healthier, more realistic acceptance of themselves, their handicap, their limitations, and their strengths. This usually happens with a good, supportive family unit and later, with understanding peers.

REFERENCES

1. Oettinger, K.: "Normal Adolescence." New York: Scribner Library, 1968.
2. Friedman, R. S.: Modeling behavior of nondisabled and disabled adolescent based upon social preference for and similarity to nondisabled and disabled models. Ph.D. dissertation. Hofstra University, Hempstead, Long Island, N.Y., 1974.
3. Waldhorn, H. K.: "Rehabilitation of the Physically Handicapped Adolescent." New York: John Day, 1972.
4. Martin, H. P.: Parental response to handicapped children. Dev. Med. Child Neurol. 17:251–252, 1975.
5. Richmond, J. B.: The family and the handicapped child. Clinical Proceedings, Children's Hospital National Medical Center. 29:156–164, 1973.
6. Caplan, G., and Lebovivi, S.: "Adolescence: Psychosocial Perspective." New York: Basic Books, 1969.
7. Brutten, M., Richardson, S., and Mangel, C.: "Something's Wrong With My Child." New York: Harcourt, Brace & Jovanovich, 1973.
8. Freeman, R. D.: Psychiatric problems in adolescents with cerebral palsy. Dev. Med. Child Neurol. 12:64, 1970.
9. Dorner, S.: Psychological and social problems of families of adolescent spina bifida patients: A preliminary report. Dev. Med. Child Neurol. (Suppl.) 29:24–26, 1973.
10. Centers, L., and Centers, R.: Peer group attitudes toward the amputee child. J. Soc. Psychol. 61:127–131, 1963.
11. Tringo, J.: The hierarchy of preference toward disability groups. J. Special Ed. 4:295–306, 1970.

12. Yuker, H. E., Block, J. R., and Younng, J. H.: "The Measurement of Attitudes Toward Disabled Persons." New York: Albertson, 1970.
13. Schooler, J. C., (ed.): "Current Issues in Adolescent Psychiatry." New York: Brunner-Mazel, 1973.
14. Seidel, U. P., Chadwick, O. F. D., and Rutter, M.: Psychological disorders in crippled children. A comparative study of children with and without brain damage. Dev. Med. Child Neurol. 17:563–573, 1975.
15. Grinberg, L., and Grinberg, R.: Pathological aspects of identity in adolescence. Contemporary Psychoanalysis. 10:27–40, 1974.
16. Blaine, G. B., Jr.: Meeting the challenge of today's adolescent. Del. Med. J. 45:193–196, 1973.
17. Williams, S. S.: Alienation of youth as reflected in the hippie movement. J. Am. Acad. Child Psychol. 9:251, 1970.
18. Dorner, S.: The relationship of physical handicap to stress in families with an adolescent with spina bifida. Dev. Med. Child Neurol. 17:765–776, 1975.

III
INDIVIDUAL AND FAMILY NEEDS

On Deciding the Use of the Family Commons

Raymond S. Duff, MD, MPH

Professional intervention for decision making and psychologic support in the situation of the handicapped child may be examined in terms of the use of resources such as economic, human, material, and technical. Following Hardin's notion, we may say there is a *societal* commons, that collection of all resources available for use by a given society [1]. Within societal commons, there are several subsets. Hiatt named one of these the *medical* commons, those resources set aside for care of sick people and for preventive services [2]. The *family* may also be said to have a commons, those limited, private resources on which individuals and their families depend and must protect in order to function or even to survive.

One of the properties of any commons is that resources rarely, if ever, are sufficient to meet demands; a second is that there is no technical solution to this problem. To cope with these difficulties, those in each commons quite naturally seek to expand their resources and to allocate all of them with care. Governments may annex or subdue those beyond their borders; may press individuals or institutions within to be more productive; or in the case of health services, may order those responsible for the medical or family commons through taxes or other means to dispose of their resources in particular ways. Those in charge of the medical commons may make attempts to be more productive or to expand by claiming more resources from societal or family commons. Families may behave similarly toward societal or medical commons. Since decisions for care of the sick are made in this field of competing interests, the distribution of power among those deciding care and the decision rules they follow are critical issues. An examination of the situation in which the care of handicapped infants is decided may be instructive.

The birth of a child is a deeply moving experience, especially for the family. If healthy, the parents usually rejoice for their happy dreams are materializing, their fears of misfortune receding. They share a joint venture of re-creating themselves and look forward to a good future. The grandparents are elated, for their children's success is also their own. They can feel freer to live, for now they have more daring to die because part of themselves reaches into yet another generation. A sense of immortality is felt, and it is good. In the delivery room, the announcement that the baby appears normal and is doing well is received with dramatic relief. People look comfortably into each other's eyes and often smile. Parents may weep with joy. The family can celebrate the arrival of a new member and life goes on.

If the baby is in trouble, the feelings of all are in turmoil. Typically, the parents are gripped by the fear that they have done a bad job, that their frightening dreams are coming true. But they also ride on the momentum of their fondest hopes and look for signals that the bad news is not really so bad. The piercing looks of their eyes are withering, and others who dare to look back at them turn away first. The parents do not know whether to listen or what to say. They fear hearing bad news and dread sharing this news with each other, the grandparents, and other family members. To care for the baby and mother, the doctors and nurses may be very busy and that usually is appropriate, or they may become conveniently busy and perhaps remain so indefinitely to evade the impact of the drama upon themselves. Herein lies a major dilemma in the whole process of deciding care and providing support. Within moments following birth, parents may feel not only sorrow for their misfortune but agonizing loneliness and bewilderment as well. Presumably powerful people, able experts in the diagnosis and treatment of diseases, often cannot tell parents the truth because they (the professionals) cannot bear to share the sorrow of it. From the parents' viewpoint, that can be the most sorrowful truth of all; for then, they may lose confidence that they can face the tragedy themselves. Their withering looks may be turned inward, and they may even lose the capacity to share with each other despite previous successes in doing so. They feel impotent.

While professionals may feel impotent in the face of problems they know they cannot solve, they may cover that up with a display of efficient professionalism. Parents may sense that and feel there is fraud in it. However, they rarely test this because they hope the implied promises of this professionalism can be fulfilled and because they have a vague mistrust of the ability of the professionals to understand their travail. That travail often is aggravated by an unspoken wish for the child's death if full recovery is impossible. As a result, the hopes of parents and professionals alike are placed largely on the technology of medicine whether or not this makes sense. The decisions which follow may have several consequences. Technology may be exploited for the child's interests, or the family may feel that it and the child are exploited for the advancement of technology. While the truth usually lies closer to the former, lack of candor in the professional-parent relationship favors technologic and hence professional dominance.

If technology succeeds, all is well, but it cannot succeed fully by definition in the case of handicapped persons. Fox [3] describes prevalent family feelings in such situations. First there is no one available to relate to and negotiate with the family. One parent reported, "We need one person, someone who could come to us or we could go to him, and he'd have time to talk to us and the knowledge we need." Second, regarding concrete suggestions and guidance in dealing with the vexing problems of handicapped persons, Fox writes, "Often the parents felt fobbed off with pity they could not use." Quoting another parent, he adds, "You can just see them humoring you; it's no good, sympathy without action." Third, medical decisions binding upon child and family alike are made without suitable regard for either, particularly as viewed by the family. One family noted, "Wonderful, they've saved another life. But they don't get the back-lash, we're the ones who have to take them over at home. I think they're hypocrites, all of them" [3]. Such sentiments are more than anecdotal. Families into which handicapped children are born become handicapped more often than do control families [4].

Professional dominance of decision making has strong support outside medicine because society has accepted a broad definition of morbidity and has created a crusading ethic to defeat disease and death by the development and application of medical technology. Voluntary health agencies representing various disease categories are the sources of much propaganda for public support. Medical technology itself often provides the basis for publicity because it can claim some spectacular successes. It is improving, more promising discoveries are appearing, and practically no one seeks the return of technologic innocence.

The use of medical technology is encouraged in hospitals for additional reasons. Especially at the end of life when technology is largely ineffective, very costly, and often dehumanizing, it may be used chiefly because physicians and families fear being charged with neglect of patients or even with homicide if death occurs as the result of less-than-heroic treatment. It is easy to understand why we say that clergymen counsel, lawyers advise, and doctors order. Doctors, it is contended, must have such authority in order to accomplish their mission or to stay out of trouble.

Several problems arise from such professional dominance of decision making. Since the basic methods of technology are reductionistic (there being no other choice), the mysteries of parts and processes are the primary focus of attention while persons, families, and the public plus the interests they hold are kept in the background. There is real danger that the holders of technology's "mysteries" may dictate both patient care and public policy [5]. In the name of justice for the sick or handicapped individual or in keeping with one reasonably comfortable doctrine or another, the medical profession and related organizations have restricted the autonomy of individuals and families. In effect, they often have assaulted both by holding that treating diseases in ways they choose is right, that treating diseases is the same as caring for those who have them, and that families and the public must support such treatment. Using the reductionistic approach to problem solving, physicians may overlook issues of morality and equity because understanding these requires a different kind of analysis [6], the performance of which the profession believes would obstruct the mission it thinks the public has given to it. Obviously, there are several assumptions here which should be questioned, but the profession is more likely to assert, "Never mind philosophizing, we are here to save lives."

In earlier work with adults [7] and later with children [8], we encountered numerous instances of physicians deciding unilaterally to carry out diagnostic, treatment, or life-extending procedures without considering the morality or equity of their choices and without achieving anything resembling informed consent by the persons or families most involved. Understandably, this was mostly the result of urgency of clinical situations or of sick persons and their families preferring to depend upon the profession and to trust its judgment in the management of individual illnesses. Although the profession sometimes may have served its own interests (such as economic or advancement of the state of the art), it is probable that most physicians did what they believed was correct for individual patients. Also, they felt that patients and families agreed with them.

This approach to medical decision making has been associated with spectacular growth of the medical commons — a two- to three-fold increase in terms of gross national product during the past 30 years — and the growth continues. We now have a vast medical-industrial complex which serves the people, but to maintain itself and to advance its cause, it also must exploit patient, family, and societal resources [9]. While the growth of the medical commons has been great, there is doubt whether significant changes in morbidity or mortality rates have always resulted [10]. There is also doubt whether the dehumanizing costs of technology have been given sufficient consideration. Both patients and families may suffer for minimal gains or none at all. A two-part question is asked here: at what point do doctors become servants of technology instead of helpers of people, supporters of unexamined doctrines rather than healers of the sick?

A POSSIBLE APPROACH

Many members of the medical profession recognize these problems. Indeed, the profession claims a long tradition of using "clinical judgment" to cope with them. In the case of teams of health professionals trying to serve the interests of individuals and families, this, ideally, involves a *process* of decision making in which persons attempt to adapt to complex and often tragic situations of life and death. Several features of this process are recognized. First, physicians are experts in the arts of diagnosis, treatment, and prognosis of diseases. Their knowledge and skills are essential to guide patient care. Second, nurses, social workers, and appropriate other staff are also commonly concerned with deciding and carrying out patient care. In some situations, their decisions, skills and support are more important than are those of the physician. Third, the patient and his family are always participants in decision making. Assisted often by social workers, nurses, and sometimes others, patients and families help physicians decide which choices will protect the most cherished values of intimately involved persons. Patients (when able), families, and health professionals puzzle at length over clinical problems, family and social situations, resources, options, values, risks, and expected results. They do this because the implications of their decisions are far reaching. At issue are how family and other resources are used, how people live, and even at times how and when they die. Since individuals have strong feelings about such things, the deliberated choices of patients and families should be considered pivotal if not paramount for they primarily must bear the consequences.

This general approach to decision making in complex situations has been illuminated by scholars from several disciplines, for example, Fletcher [11], from ethics, and Bickel [12], from law. More elaborate work from political science and economics has been done on decision making by Lindblom, who describes the essential steps of "muddling through" when other ways of deciding fail [13]. Braybrooke and Lindblom [14], the former a philosopher, contend that strategies for policy evaluation and decision making should reflect the ways persons think about problems and the nature of the problems themselves. About thinking, they wrote:

> When a man sets out to solve a problem, he embarks on a course of mental activity more circuitous, more complex, more subtle, and perhaps more idiosyncratic than he perceives. If he is aware of some of the grosser aspects of his own problem solving, as when he consciously focuses his attention on what he has identified as a critical unknown, he will often have only the feeblest insight into how his mind finds, creates, dredges up — which of these he does not know — a new idea. Dodging in and out of the unconscious, moving back and forth from concrete to abstract, trying chance here and system there, soaring, jumping, backtracking, crawling, sometimes freezing on point like a bird dog, he exploits mental processes that are only slowly yielding to observation and systematic description.

When this thinking is applied to complex problems in a strategy they call "incrementalism," some mutually reinforcing adaptations comprising a system of analysis emerge. This incrementalism "holds that the problem of evaluation is simplified by a concentration on social evils rather than on utopias; that limits on man's competence are acknowledged in reforms that alter only relatively small parts of the social structure at any one time; that continuity in readjustment diminishes the need to be right in any single decision; that aims change with experience with policy; and that experiments in social reform teach some things that cannot be learned in any other way."

Note how applicable these notions are to clinical medicine. We seek to solve all problems of illness and escape death. But this utopia (or perhaps nightmare) being impossible, we deal with what is manageable. We often propose actions requiring vast family or social reforms which cannot or will not occur. So, we make adjustments. In caring for patients, we make many decisions some of which, including major ones, we know will be wrong when examined in retrospect. We will change as we learn from these mistakes. For some problems, the only other approach is paralysis.

This process of decision making reflects the vastly varied realities it addresses. It permits a more or less systematic approach to personal, family, or social issues which usually cannot be evaluated or resolved by the rules of ideals, the dictates of doctrines, or deductive analyses. The process is pragmatic, democratic, conservative, continuous, and untidy. It is based on ethical relativism and demands consistent, thoughtful skepticism. It probably requires a good measure of faith, and since altruism at least within the family is almost certainly built into our genes, that faith is probably justified [15]. While the tormenting perplexities of deciding in this way may drive many to the rules of one doctrine or another, these are unworkable here. They hinder analysis, silence protest, and ensure the tyranny of some (even a small minority) over others. Because values are often fluid and may be in conflict with one another, the most cherished ones recognizable in a particular situation may be imperiled if the process yields to another way. Parochial or dogmatic views and the values they represent are important and always must be given recognition when patients or families hold them in particular situations. Failure to do this would be inconsistent with ethical relativism. However, no view or value is consistently supreme over all others all of the time. Thus, some values will be ignored or lost. Sometimes, outright sacrifices, even large ones, are made. Since there is no escape from some tragic choices, tension and controversy are inevitable.

Some physicians, for example, Beeson [16], believe that families should not be asked to share decision making as described here. For then, family guilt feelings would be increased, and this would add to their already existing burdens of dealing with illness and tragedy. Also, families may be incapable of understanding the issues well enough to make reasoned decisions. At times there are difficulties here because some persons have no families or because some families will fail to help. However, physicians commonly underestimate lay knowledge and perhaps lay abilities to learn. The knowledge gap is more in the perception of the physician than in the reality [17]. In our experiences, sharing decision making does things for families which may not be immediately apparent. Such sharing implies that health professionals believe families can and should help to make decisions and can be trusted to formulate good and just choices. This gives families a good feeling, a vote of confidence. They need and deserve a sense of control and independence which they get from it. They commonly respond with great efforts which are of a high, even sacred, order in their value system and in society's. Families usually feel those who love and care the most will also grieve and agonize more than anyone over illness, handicap, and other tragedies. From years of dealings with families, it appears to us that those who share decision making generally understand the issues well, make difficult choices as well as anyone else and often better, are close to and supported by health professionals, support and teach health professionals a great deal, and recover from their trials sooner. In working with social workers, nurses, and others, such families can reform services and thus obviate the difficulties described by Fox [3]. Patients and families achieve some order of control despite great losses and confusion and thus blunt or escape the destructive impact of feelings of helplessness. They may even become stronger because of their trials [18].

Some recurring questions in deciding the care of handicapped children illustrate this process of decision making. It is generally agreed that life is a great value to all. But particular persons in some situations may place freedom from suffering and severe incapacity above it. Accordingly, it is reasonable at times to choose death for the sake of the individual. For the well-being of the unfortunate most persons believe the more fortunate at the moment should sacrifice at least to the extent they would want others to sacrifice when misfortune strikes them. This reciprocal relationship is adaptive. It ensures survival of individuals through cooperation. But its application is difficult. Intense ambivalence is inevitable because the relationship often involves choosing between altruism and selfishness. There are times, for example, when one must decide between the well-being of the unfortunate and that of others in competition for limited resources. By direct or proxy decision, it may be reasonable at times to make a tragic choice of neglect, even death, for one in order to protect others. To be nurtured, protected, and oriented to life by a secure and loving family is a great value. Then, given the capacity to benefit from this, one may achieve a healthy sense of self-esteem and the ability to relate intimately and comfortably with others. But if a person cannot benefit from this or if attempts to provide it destroy greater values held by other family members, the choice may be foolish. If the family is badly damaged or destroyed, this value will be lost along with many additional values held by all family members. Hence, it is reasonable at times to make a tragic choice of placing an individual outside the home — a partial social death from the individual and family viewpoints. A foster family may be preferred to an institution because institutions generally have done poorly as a substitute for the family. But how will a child fare and how will the foster family make out? Various choices may be selected here. Treatment to limit handicaps and to restore function may be preferred to no treatment. But most treatments are costly and some are inhumane. Moreover, they may provide only marginal benefits or be harmful.

Other services, including disease prevention, education, and housing may be more valuable in controlling family and societal morbidity and mortality rates. Thus, there are conflicts between or among patient, family, and society. While the resolution of such conflicts by reductionistic analysis fails, the *process* of deciding by incrementalism offers some help.

If we can reasonably put our faith in this process of deciding care, the birth of a handicapped child should be followed by systematic exploration of several topics. First, the nature of the child's problem should be assessed. Available management schemes and the respective costs (economic and human) and benefits should be articulated. Parents should be fully informed in ways that make sense to them. The degree of uncertainty about diagnosis, treatment, and prognosis should be discussed. Second, the nature of the family, particularly the unique ways they perceive and may adapt to the situation, should be evaluated. Parents should be told that the best decisions for any child and family probably will arise from an exchange of views and observations between health professionals and the family regarding the child's condition, family realities, and what is possible or practical to do. Various choices which other families and health professionals have made under similar circumstances may be reviewed along with new choices which seem reasonable to the persons deciding care. In brief, deciding the care and management of children with handicaps should be done in full recognition of social as well as disease and treatment realities.

If this is done, the process of deciding care will necessarily provide for a great deal of psychologic support, perhaps maximal support. Families and health professionals will come to understand each other well because their relationship will necessarily be intense. Social distance is short — a major achievement in a situation where it is usually long because professionals, often being held in high esteem, are removed from most citizens. Lemkau [19] emphasizes the importance of short social distances for helping people in trouble. This relationship probably better than any other permits the parties in it to make decisions based on strengths rather than on weaknesses because both will have been identified. That should enhance adaptation based primarily on family initiatives. According to Pless et al [20] and our own observations, families generally have found that professionals despite their claims have no substitutes. Patients and families are the chief persons who must cope with illness and handicaps.

Regarding the use of resources, health professionals should make clear that often these must be rationed at one level or another because there is a gap between resources and demands. As a result of further advances in medicine, this gap almost certainly will become a gulf. Families ought to be given a chance to understand such issues, especially because the family commons is often endangered, along with the medical commons, by the decisions that are made [2]. A curious, perhaps fortuitous, paradox should be noted here: the most expensive services are often the least valuable [21]. Citizens who understand the propaganda of crusaders as well as the unique and valuable services they provide have a chance to maximize benefits while protecting family resources.

This policy of deciding care may displease some health professionals and those in the health industry who profit from providing services. Also, it may displease those who are watchdogs for various moral views. But it may be better for patients and families and for society as a whole.

While the specifics of dealing with families of handicapped children are extremely varied and often are unique to the families and the health professionals involved, a few general guides have stood out in our experience. These will be summarized.

There is no substitute for truth telling which must be adhered to by health professionals and families so that the medical and social realities may be confronted. Families almost never complain when they are told what they must eventually face in any case. On the other hand, they often feel confused, resentful, and put down if important news is withheld from them or if professionals do not absorb and ponder what they have to say.

Most families are more resilient than health professionals believe. It is safe, even preferable, to encourage infant-parent [22] and at times infant-sib contact. All requests for information and for physical encounters between family members and the infant should be respected and usually honored. This is generally true regardless of the severity of the problem, the degree of the infant's ugliness, or the prognosis. In our experience, parents in specific situations have been shown their infants, live, dying, or dead and with diverse deformities, including anencephaly. They have felt, held, and talked with such infants. They may grieve the misfortune and curse its falling on them, or they may see in the infant chiefly the things which are normal and good and thank God for an experience which brought them closer together. Their reactions are as varied as they themselves. Failure to encourage such an approach usually leaves families isolated with fantasies more ugly than the reality. Then, they cannot join with one another or with health professionals to decide whether to give up on a cause which is probably lost or to act realistically in concert to restore, rehabilitate, and make the best of their misfortune. They may live by fiction and waste resources. They may grieve ineffectively and fail to share with one another the joys or the sorrows of the occasion. Their existing children, if any, may drift into major, long-lasting psychologic difficulties.

The final choice of care should represent the synthesis of social and medical data in that order. As Sigerist [23] notes, the aims of medicine are social. Depending on the situation, the doctor or other health professionals, such as a nurse or a social worker, may be the chief person to help the family decide care and live with the consequences. While the physician will have to bear the final medical responsibility, the contributions of others to resolving questions of care must always be taken into account. Physicians are not so godlike that they can or should decide and act alone in situations where there are respected divisions of opinion about the ethics of available medical choices. If a particular physician finds a family choice personally objectionable, he should so indicate and perhaps withdraw as he recruits another physician having more cosmopolitan views. The medical profession rightly belongs more to families and the public than to itself [24]. The same reasoning applies to other health professionals.

Professionals probably should come to understand the pleas of families in trouble in the following ways. While we as families may adhere to absolutist views in many things most of the time for this is comforting, do not expect us to live by them always. Be reluctant to make decisions which seriously deplete or destroy our commons whether these are based on your personal dogmatism or even our own. For then, while we may have perfection by some rule, ironically, we may achieve a perfect injustice and be oppressed by its tyranny. Rather, help us to understand the nature of the tragedy we face. Let us discuss the potentials and limits which we and you have to cope with tragedy. Help us to appreciate that misguided altruism can be as ruinous as selfishness and that selfishness despite its bad name may sometimes be a superior moral choice. After all, altruism *is* selfishness when the first and second persons are reversed. Then, let us decide together what makes most sense in our tragedy: great efforts for physical and social rehabilitation, limited efforts for either or both of these, or a loving, sorrowful consignment to the grave. This last choice should be available if necessary to escape brutal diseases on the one hand or the inhumanities of largely useless treatment on the other [25, 26]. In any case, until we die, let us keep an open, contemplative mind and from time to time change our course according to changing conditions. This will permit us to adapt: to find and use our greatest strengths for our handicapped and ourselves. It will give us an imperfect justice, not utopia, but that is all we can expect.

These issues are rooted deeply in society. While individuals may describe them, society will have to look to itself for the solution. Failing that, a tyranny of rules and the power of a few will dominate and often destroy families; with that, the well-being and sometimes the lives of many more individuals besides the sick and the handicapped will be sacrificed. The ironies of the crusade against disease must be averted if the crusade is to be most effective. One way to do this is to grant patients and families the autonomy to protect the family commons by placing adaptation above the drive for utopia or even fairness when in their view there is no reasonable alternative. This would establish a family-centered ethical principle which acknowledges the vast complexities and the incredible unfairness which have characterized our biologic and social evolution. Such "ecologized" ethics may appear brutal. But they may be kind and just, for in using them individuals and families assisted by health professionals may reduce the hypocrisies and tyrannies of the present, fulfill their promises to one another, and decide a prudent course for present and future generations.

REFERENCES

1. Hardin, G.: The tragedy of the commons. Science 162:1243–1248, 1968.
2. Hiatt, H. H.: Protecting the medical commons: Who is responsible?, N. Engl. J. Med. 293:235–241, 1975.
3. Editorial: The handicapped family. Lancet 2:400–401, 1975.
4. Tew, B. J., Pazno, H., and Laurence, K. M.: Must a family with a handicapped child be a handicapped family? Dev. Med. Child Neurol. (Suppl. 32) 16:95–98, 1974.
5. Mahler, H.: Health – A demystification of medical technology. Lancet 2:829–833, 1975.
6. Frank, J. D.: "Persuasion and Healing," Rev. Ed. New York: Schocken Books, 1974.
7. Duff, R. S., and Hollinghead, A. B.: "Sickness and Society." New York: Harper and Row, 1968.
8. Duff, R. S., and Campbell, A. G. M.: Moral and ethical dilemmas in the special care nursery. N. Engl. J. Med. 289:894, 1973.
9. Waitzkin, H. B., and Waterman, B.: "The Exploitation of Illness in Capitalist Society." New York: The Bobbs-Merrill Company, 1974.
10. NcNerney, W. J.: Health care reforms – The myths and realities. Am. J. Public Health 61:222–232, 1971.
11. Fletcher, J.: "Situation Ethics, The New Morality." Philadelphia: The Westminster Press, 1966.
12. Bickel, A. M.: "The Morality of Consent." New Haven: Yale University Press, 1975.
13. Lindblom, C. E.: The science of "muddling through." Public Administration Review 19:79–88, 1959.
14. Braybrooke, D. and Lindblom, C. E.: "A Strategy of Decision, Policy Evaluation as a Social Process." New York: The Free Press, 1970.
15. Wilson, E. O.: "Sociobiology, The New Synthesis." Cambridge: The Belknap Press of Harvard University Press, 1975.
16. Beeson, P. B.: Quality of survival. In McLachlan, G. (Ed.): "Patient, Doctor Society, A Symposium of Introspection." London: Oxford University Press, 1972.
17. McKinlay, T. B.: Who is really ignorant – physician or patient? J. Health Soc. Behav. 16:3–11, 1975.
18. Seligman, M. E. P.: "Helplessness: On Depression, Development, and Death." San Francisco: W. H. Freeman and Company, 1975.
19. Lemkau, P. V.: "Mental Hygiene in Public Health," 2nd Ed. New York: McGraw-Hill, 1955.
20. Haggerty, R. J., Roghman, K. J., and Pless, I. B.: "Child Health and the Community." New York: John Wiley & Sons, 1975.
21. Thomas, L.: Reflections on the science and technology of medicine. Yale Medicine, 8:1, 1973.

22. Kennell, J. H., Jerauld, R., Wolfe, H., Chesler, D., Kreger, N. C., McAlpine, W., Steffa, M. and Klaus, M.: Maternal behavior one year after early and extended post-partum contact. Dev. Med. Child Neurol. 16:172–179, 1974.
23. Sigerist, H. E.: "A History of Medicine." New York: Oxford University Press, 1951.
24. Page, B. B.: Who "owns" the professions? The Hastings Center Report 5 (5), 1975.
25. Jonsen, A. R., Phibbs, R. H., Tonley, W. H., and Garland, M. J.: Critical issues in newborn intensive care. Pediatrics 55:756–768, 1975.
26. Duff, R. S., and Campbell, A. G. M.: On deciding the care of severely handicapped or dying persons. Pediatrics 57:487–493, 1976.

Obstacles to Providing Psychologic Services to Disabled Children and Their Families

Albert J. Solnit, MD

INTRODUCTION

Children are born helpless. Without the care of a committed, affectionate adult they do not survive. Recently in London, a young unwed mother died suddenly at home of what appeared to be the rupture of a congenital aneurysm. Her healthy infant child died of starvation because no one knew the mother had died.

When a child is born, he or she enters into a world prepared to care for a healthy, intact, helpless child. By his or her responses and development, the healthy newborn reassures the family (ie parents, sibs, grandparents and others) that they are biologically intact. The child's growth and development can steadily provide evidence of parents' competence and of the strength of their inheritance, implying a promising future. Usually, the community is prepared to provide the support and services necessary for a healthy newborn child.

When a young child is developmentally disabled or has a congenital or inherited deficit, the parents feel injured. Mourning reactions of the parents require time and support in order to enable the parents to prepare for the care of the child they did not expect. Such time and support is often not available. This tends to start a downward spiral in which the average environment, one not prepared for a disabled child, becomes an environment at risk for that child and his parents.

At the same time, sibs feel threatened by uncertainty, by the further withdrawal of their parents' attention and by the fear that their own future physical and social well-being is jeopardized. In the newborn period, these challenges usually find the mother and father, but especially the mother, particularly vulnerable to what is felt as a catastrophe. Thus, there is a good deal of reason to assume that the physical disability of the child tends to be elaborated emotionally by the initial responses of parents and other members of the family, who are traumatized by the birth or development of a deviant child. Defects evoke weakness before they evoke strength.

A similar case can be made in regard to many physicians, nurses, social workers, and others who feel threatened by the birth or development of a defective child. They are likely to feel that their competence has been undermined by the failure of the child to be born and grow in a healthy manner. Additionally, they often feel discomforted by their inability to make precise forecasts, or to provide clear explanations of what has happened to bring about the condition.

Therefore, in general, obstacles to the care of the developmentally disabled child are fundamentally related to the dynamic equation that health brings acceptance and support whereas disability evokes an increasing risk in an environment that is organized for the able or healthy child. One of the major expressions of these dynamic relationships is the reactive tendency for a family with healthy, resilient relationships to mobilize its resources to master the challenge; whereas the troubled, underprivileged or disadvantaged family becomes all the more unable to cope when a defective or disabled child becomes a member of their family. Two other concrete examples can illustrate how defect evokes weakness and how health evokes confidence and competence.

Professionals are more likely to righteously impose services in the care of a disabled child if they feel the family has not responded as the physician, nurse, or social worker feel they should. Thus, the defensive reactions of professionals tend to discourage a family's self-help attitudes and to interefere with the development of a therapeutic alliance between the family and the health workers. That is, while the family is still absorbing the experience of having a disabled child, the professionals often respond initially to their own urge to master the challenge of the child's disability and are not in touch with the family's mourning and coping reactions.

The complexity and scarcity of multidisciplinary services make it very difficult for parents to discover how to enter the system of services that are available, leaving such parents with a magnified sense of helplessness and hopelessness.

Finally, our limitations in organizing and coordinating multidisciplinary services are a painful indicator that our ability to understand and treat specific aspects of a disability in a child has far outstripped our capacity to orchestrate all the aspects of diagnostic and therapeutic-rehabilitation services that our knowledge tells us is — or should be — available for disabled children and their families. It is this final point that impelled Dr. Ronald MacKeith to write in 1969 under the title, "The Buck Stops." "The care of the handicapped goes on for a long time and is usually complex, at first medically and later educationally and then vocationally, with medical, psychiatric and social issues playing larger or smaller parts at various periods. . . . Some one person has to feel responsible and the various agents involved have to accept him as their coordinator. . . . This is not to take responsibility away from parents or from other professional people involved."*

---

*In "Developmental Medicine and Child Neurology," Dec. 1969, vol. II, no. 6, pp. 691–693.

THREE OBSTACLES

There are three large categories of problems in developing mental health services for children. The first is the role of children in our society, one in which their rights and priorities are usually pushed aside in favor of the needs of the adults. This can be understood in a number of ways, including the historic and current obstacles to achieving an improvement of the actual status of children in competition with adults for limited resources. These priorities are especially evident in regard to mental health services and in providing for psychologic aspects of the care of the handicapped or developmentally disabled child.

As the structure and function of the family has changed over the years, we have become aware that each parent is expected to attach himself emotionally to his children as intimate members of his household for 16 or 18 years, rather than 7 or 8 years as was the case in the Middle Ages. In the case of a family with a disabled child, those prolonged attachments are complex and usually more highly conflicted. The resolution of these conflicts determines the outcome of these attachments.

Now, each parent can invest more in each child as a carrier of his aspirations for the future. Our increased psychologic understanding reveals that in the family as we know it children have come to represent both our replacements and our hopes for immortality. These representations are both powerful and ambivalent, having a potential range from the most intense love to the most fearful resentment. Thus, the ambivalent psychologic roots and complexities of parents who serve as advocate for their children have deepened and elaborated in the contemporary family with all of its vicissitudes. The disabled child heightens this ambivalence because the increased negative feelings are unacceptable.

Why are we so unsuccessful in assuring children of a high priority in terms of an advocacy that taps into our resources, values and limited altruism? Adults have deeply ingrained, irrational reservations about the primacy of children's needs because they expect to be replaced by them. Similarly, adults have a deep love and concern for children because parents hope their children's lives will fulfill their own values and aspirations. Unwittingly, in this way, parents express their wishes for immortality and reduce their fear of death. Thus, parents universally experience children as representatives of their mortality as well as their immortality, of their weaknesses and their strengths. A disabled child complicates the conflicted feeling parents face normatively. In each culture, a certain ethnic political and social pattern of a given historic period will reflect the psychologic meaning of the disabled child to his community. This meaning, in turn, will have a marked influence on the balance of these ambivalent parental attitudes and on the priorities assigned to the societal resources provided for such children.

The second category of problems is rooted in the developmental complexities of childhood. These complexities tend to be oversimplified in attempting to find a useful and scientifically satisfactory classification of developmental deviation and mental illness in childhood; eg responding to our preference for neatness and simplification, we attempt to classify with an underlying presumption of "either/or;" ie either it is the nature of the child's physical deficit or it is the parents' and child's emotional reactions to the handicap that is emphasized. The major deficit is either physical or psychologic. In fact, it is always both. Therefore, our classification systems must be used with an awareness of the purpose of the particular system: 1) Is it to register morbidity? 2) Is it to communicate need for services? or 3) Is it meant to inventory the child's assets as well as that of the family's more than the deficits? The lack of a satisfactory classification system, a reflection of our "either/or" tendency, increases our difficulties in developing epidemiologic instruments that will enable us to know more clearly the scope and nature of what is termed developmental disabilities. According to the Developmental Disabilities Services and Facilities Construction Act, Sec. 102 (7), as amended in 1975, "The term 'developmental disability' means a disability of a person which:

"(A) (i) is attributable to mental retardation, cerebral palsy, epilepsy, or autism;
(ii) is attributable to any other condition of a person found to be closely related to mental retardation because such condition results in similar impairment of general intellectual functioning or adaptive behavior to that of mentally retarded persons or requires treatment and services similar to those required for such persons; or
(iii) is attributable to dyslexia resulting from a disability described in clause (i) or (ii) of this subparagraph;
"(B) originates before such person attains age eighteen;
"(C) has continued or can be expected to continue indefinitely; and
"(D) constitutes a substantial handicap to such person's ability to function normally in society."*

This lack of precision tends to blur our knowledge about the so-called natural course of illness and the impact of various treatment modalities. These diagnostic categories also reflect the difficulties we have in making predictions about the outcome of developmental crises and the interactions of various environmental conditions on different states of childhood and youth in disabled children. Thus, the need for improved understanding of vulnerability, risk and mastery in childhood and youth is a critical one. Labeling is necessary, but a particular system of labeling usually is intended to serve aims other than diagnosis or treatment (rehabilitation). Often the underlying reason, or reasons, is to gain political support or to minimize highly charged superstitions or fears in the community.

In our evaluations we are well advised to do balanced inventories of assets

*Developmental Disabilities Services and Facilities Construction Act, 42 USC 6001 as amended by Public Law 94-103, 94th Congress, H.R. 4005, October 4, 1975.

and liabilities and to be aware of how various classification systems serve differing aims; eg a mother is not either rejecting or not rejecting. As Anna Freud pointed out, there are no rejecting mothers. Such a label simply camouflages the complexity by a disarming simplicity.

The third large category of obstacles is that of qualified personnel. Although in a certain sense this completes the circle by connecting with the problem of inadequate priorities for children, it also has historic roots in the several disciplines — medicine, nursing, social work, education and psychology — whose knowledge and skills are necessary to serve disabled children and their families. The desirable and necessary dependency of the child explains why the decision to seek assistance rests with the parents and why the services are often provided indirectly through the parents as well as directly to the child. The full discussion of the disabled child's needs and how they impinge on the family as well as on the family's place in the community will further indicate why physiotherapists, pediatricians, psychiatrists, psychologists, neurologists, surgeons, social workers, nurses, teachers and others have collaborated in providing a full array of services for disabled children. This complicates the manpower shortage at the same time as it increases the flexibility in developing manpower for such services. The rationale, for having a multidisciplinary team to provide services for disabled children and their families can also be explained by saying that society has increasingly expected and prepared adults other than the parents to play a vital role in the care, guidance and protection of the growing child, disabled or not.

In fact, as has already been suggested, we are relatively incompetent in orchestrating the services of a multidisciplinary group. The failure of such an orchestration can be viewed as the risks of dehumanization, failure of coordination and a breakdown of the continuity of the necessary services sought by the parents for their child. For similar reasons, we are also inferior in any effort at long-term planning for needed human services.

The psychology of our technologic society moves toward the assumption that manpower and knowledge can be produced instantly if financial support is offered. Finances by themselves do not provide sufficient stimulus or support to assure the availability of competent services. In fact, financial support tied to a demand for immediate services without lead time to train personnel is likely to invite a lowering of standards by cutting back on manpower qualifications and reducing the quality of the care offered in order to fit the manpower that is available.

It would be more appropriate and effective if we could grit our teeth for a preparatory period in which we educate and train adequate personnel — adequate in qualifications and numbers — to meet the challenge of carrying out a complex task competently and tactfully. If we lower the standards of assessment and care to fit the personnel available, we subscribe to inferior services for developmentally disabled children and their families.

CONCLUSION

There is much to be said for the inspiring ways in which children and parents meet the challenge of disabilities by unfolding and activating resources that enable the child to master or compensate for his deficit in a developmentally progressive way. Resiliency, practice and innovation can lead to increasing mastery and in many instances to compensatory responses that culminate in the acquisition of talent and the uncovering of creativity.

Families confront many difficulties and obstacles in their efforts to help their handicapped children by finding the diagnostic, therapeutic and rehabilitative services and the community supports that are necessary for rehabilitation and mastery. These families are in urgent need of access to sustained community services in order to ward off the downward spiral in which the initial disability enlarges and becomes the basis for arrested development. There is reason to believe that the challenge of an initial disability can often become the basis for an upward spiral, the sweet music of compensatory reactions and the achievement of mastery that leads to a progressive development.

Our great hope is for the development of services that are so attractive, usable and available that parents will know how to find them and will voluntarily seek them out and exploit them. In this way the obstacles can be overcome because parents will know how to enter, utilize and leave the system of services for their children and families when defect, disability, and handicap are associated with the beginning of life.

In summary, weakness and defects in infancy tend to evoke the psychologic risks in the environment more commonly than they evoke compensatory psychologic and emotional resources in the family.

When the weak or defective child evokes the risks of the environment, he or she is a vulnerable or handicapped child. Less commonly, weaknesses are met by resources in the family and community that lead to mastery of the deficit and to a progressive development. Deficits and vulnerabilities can be transformed into strengths. The mental health professions can provide collaborative energies and leadership in establishing and maintaining psychologic environments that are supportive in helping each disabled child and his parents to convert weaknesses and deficits into compensatory responses and potential strengths into competencies and talents.

The priorities of children in our society, the complexity of human development and the limitations of our capacities to plan for and coordinate multidisciplinary services for children and their families are challenges that confront us. How we meet these challenging opportunities provides a substantial future view of our society.

Individual and Family Needs in the Health Care of Children With Developmental Disorders

Ivan B. Pless, MD, FRCP (C)

The term "developmental disorder" is similar in many respects to the often misused term "handicapped." Any child with a chronic physical or mental condition may be handicapped when he or she participates in an activity involving the use of an impaired organ. Similarly, children with any prolonged physical disorder may also have their development affected physically, socially, emotionally, or intellectually. Although this is a somewhat broader definition of developmental disorder than that which is used by others, it is nevertheless, a useful and important concept and one which has been validated empirically. Furthermore, when we come to examine the medical care provided for children with either type of developmental disability — those narrowly defined or those falling into the broader definition as used in this paper — it is noteworthy how similar the patterns of care prove to be.

In both instances one outstanding problem emerges: each category of disability has primary and secondary consequences which, in varying degrees, pediatricians should view as preventable. To succeed in their prevention at either level, however, may require an approach to health care quite different from that which is currently in vogue.

One challenge this problem poses for both health planners and clinicians is how to use our existing knowledge so that time, money, and personnel can be allocated most efficiently. Only in this way can the best services be provided for those who are most likely to profit from them. It is well known to epidemiologists that those who make the most demand on health services are not necessarily those who most require them. This is not to say that any system of health care can advocate neglect of any who request help. But it does suggest that more effort must be invested in distinguishing between those who are at "high risk" for a particular problem, in this case secondary developmental disorders, and those for whom the risk is significantly less.

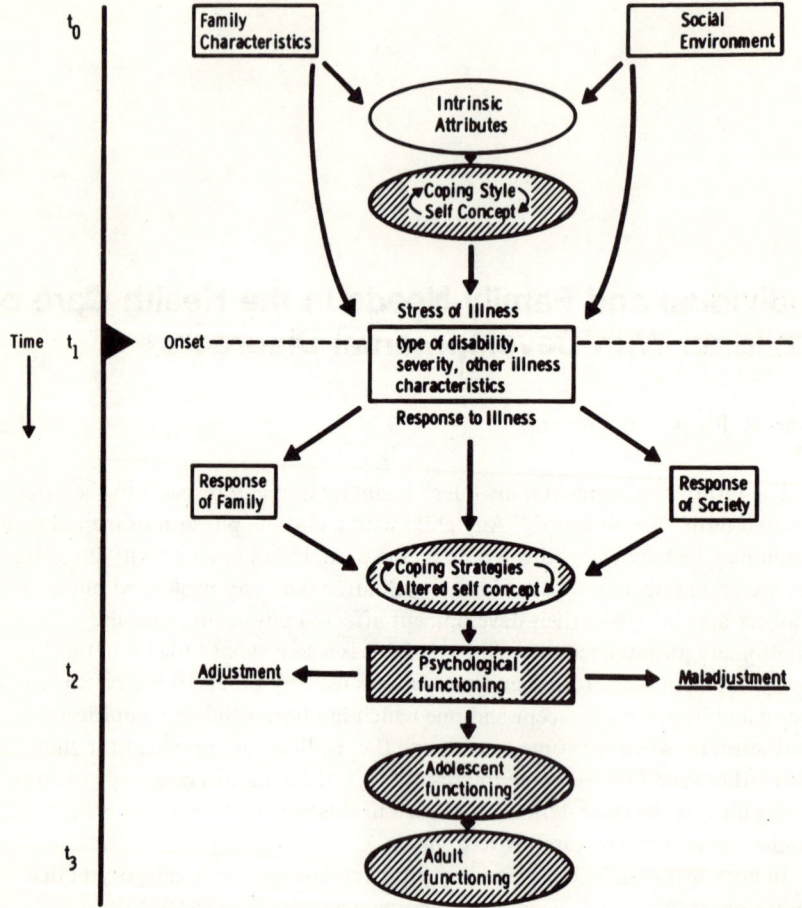

Fig. 1. The concept of adjustment: an integrated model of adjustment. From Pless, I. B., Roghmann, K., and Haggerty, R. J.: Chronic illness, family functioning, and psychological adjustment: a model for the allocation of preventive mental health services. Int. J. Epidemiol. 1:271–277, 1972.

Based on results obtained from the United Kingdom National Survey of Health and Development [1], from the Isle of Wight Survey [2], and from our own Rochester studies, it is conservatively estimated that 15–20% more children with chronic disorders experience significant impairments in their psychosocial development than do a comparable group of healthy children. When I began my studies in this field, I assumed that this figure would be much higher; indeed I hypothesized that most children would be adversely affected in one way or another. When we began to establish, through studies such as those mentioned above, that this was not the case, the goal of research shifted toward determining why some children are more handicapped in their development than others. The conceptual model described in Figure 1 presents an outline of what every clinician knows from experience. As Apley pointed out in his review of the book in which this model appears, it grossly oversimplifies the complexity of the interactions that exist between social, environmental, personality, and family factors, each of which may contribute to the emotional maladjustment of a physically disabled child [3]. It serves, however, to highlight the fact that among the many factors contributing to risk of maladjustment (including, for example, the type and severity of the disorder or the age at which it begins) one that might be identifiable with relative precision at an early point in time is the nature of the support available from the family. Accordingly, much of our subsequent work has been built around the family's central role — first, to confirm its importance as a risk factor and second, to develop intervention strategies based upon strengthening the family's preventive capabilities.

The purpose of this paper is to describe results from several studies that broadly depict the patterns of health care these children receive. In doing so I will try, indirectly, to show how well or how poorly such care attends to the goal of prevention — a concept so central to the work of the man we are honoring through this book. These patterns will be examined from 3 viewpoints: that of the parent, obtained through a sample of household interviews; that of the primary physician, obtained from a sample of office interviews; and one obtained from studies of children in specialty clinic settings.

DATA FROM HEALTH CARE SURVEY

Household Sample of Parent Interviews

In 1968, about 500 parents were interviewed in their own homes as part of a 1% random sample of families with children under the age of 18, residing in Monroe County, New York [4]. From this initial interview families were identified in which there were children with symptoms that seemed to signify a chronic physical disorder. The interview with the parent was repeated a year later, and a battery of psychologic tests were performed on the child. In addition, information was obtained from the child's teachers and peers. Although the major emphasis of this study was on developmental disorder of a psychosocial nature, parents were also asked about the child's medical care. The usual pattern was one where responsibilities were divided among a number of physicians. Most parents told of visits to a variety of specialists as well as fairly continuous contact with a single primary physician. However, many areas of need were described for which little help had been provided. It was often

TABLE 1. Health Status, Family Functioning, and Psychologic Maladjustment [9][a]

Chronic illness	Family function index scores		Age groups	
			6–11 years (n = 164)	12–18 years (n = 49)
Present	low (poor)		33%[b]	38%
	high (good)		24%	21%
		relative risk	1.38	1.81
Absent	low (poor)		18%	33%
	high (good)		13%	17%
		relative risk	1.38	1.94
		overall risk	2.54	2.24

[a]Reprinted with permission
[b]Rounded percentage with poor adjustment scores

difficult for parents to be specific about what they thought was missing, but it was clear that it was most often problems generally involving schooling, behavior, or family that were dealt with poorly, if at all.

In addition to the insights gained from these interviews with parents, this, the first of our studies in Monroe County, provided a rare opportunity to test the psychologic development of a random sample of chronically ill children [5]. By virtue of the study design, it was also possible to compare these psychologic test results with those obtained from a group of healthy children of similar sex, age, and social background. Taken together the psychosocial test measures provided an index of psychologic maladjustment.

As shown in Table 1, the results indicate that those with chronic illnesses in particular, those whose families score poorly according to the index of family functioning specifically designed for this study [6], were maladjusted significantly more often than healthy children in familes with high index scores. The results revealed significant deficits in scholastic performance among these children as well as in other measures of social development. In summary, this well-controlled study provides clear evidence that many children with chronic physical disorders are indeed at high risk for psychosocial maladjustment.

Having demonstrated this, however, the next objective was to determine ways in which such consequences could be prevented or minimized. As the conceptual model suggests, these children appeared to have in common (apart from the chronicity of their condition) a significant degree of impairment to their self-concept and to their ability to cope with stress. As time goes on a child with any disorder is likely to feel less worthy than his peers. This sets in motion a vicious circle of self-devaluation, poor performance, and increasingly disturbed behavior. If these basic findings are true a sound strategy for secondary prevention of maladjustment involves first, identification of high-risk families and second, some method for interrupting this sequence of psychologic events. This requires a person who can aid these children and their families in several ways: 1) help them learn how to place more emphasis on the child's assets and less on his disabilities; 2) help provide more information about the disease and the doctor's actions and intentions; 3) provide the therapeutic value of having a sympathetic listener; 4) provide practical help with everyday problems; 5) play the role of advocate by virtue of their understanding of the system of health and community services and have the ability to secure these services; 6) above all, they need someone to coordinate the many, often diverse components of the child's care.

In an effort to accomplish some of these objectives, we introduced the idea of the nonprofessional family counselor, a mature woman who had successfully raised a family and whose personality attributes and knowledge of the community provided a unique combination of talents [7]. To evaluate the effectiveness of this idea in achieving the goals described, a program was established so that the results could be evaluated experimentally. Six counselors were recruited, trained, and assigned to work for 1 year each with 8 families in which there was a child with a chronic illness. A comparison group of children with similar chronic disorders were used as controls. Psychologic test measures, repeated before and after a year of family intervention, clearly indicate the value of the counselor's work. The test scores showed that fewer of those who received such assistance became maladjusted (about 20%), while a majority of children in the control group showed psychologic deterioration (60%). This first program was initiated in 1970, and it has continued to function in one setting or another since then with a total of over 20 women having served in this capacity.

Regional Study of Primary Physicians

Unfortunately our subsequent experience with the counselor program showed that practitioners in private practice were reluctant to incorporate counselors into the office setting, chiefly for financial reasons. Consequently, it seemed important to try to determine more precisely the range of services doctors normally provide: Were we worrying for nothing? Was it correct to assume that many of the tasks performed by the family counselors were not being performed by most doctors? Was the program simply duplicating existing medical and social services? To answer these questions a random sample of general practitioners and pediatricians practicing in the 10 counties of the Genesee, New York region were selected [8]. A total of 84 physicians were interviewed in their offices. They were asked first, to estimate the number of children with chronic disorders they had in their practice; second, whether or not as a general rule they shared responsibilities for these children with specialists; and third, to describe what services they themselves provided or secured from others. The services inquired about were both technical, eg x-ray and laboratory tests, and supportive, eg social work. The results, as shown in Table 2, suggest that overall most services in both categories are not utilized by primary physicians. More importantly, there appeared to be no consistent relationship between either the type of disorder, (only 2 examples are given), the locale of the physician or his level of training, and the wide variety of practice patterns reported. (Although it is noteworthy that, overall, urban GPs had the highest percentage of "rarely" or "never" responses and rural pediatricians the lowest!)

The frequency with which these children are referred to specialists and responsibility shared with the specialist suggests to us that these findings might best be explained by the primary physician's assumption that when a child is sent to a specialist, whatever services may be required will be provided.

Specialty Clinic Studies

To determine the extent to which this belief was true, 2 subsequent studies were carried out in specialty clinics. Parents of children tested in these settings were asked who in the past year had provided each of 9 aspects of comprehensive care. These 9 areas were chosen to reflect the wide range of services needed by most handicapped children. The responses indicate that as a rule, responsibilities are divided so that well-child care and episodic illnesses are left to the primary

TABLE 2. Use of Services for Children With Cerebral Palsy and Epilepsy[a]

Type of Service	Disorder	Urban		Rural	
		GP	Ped	GP	Ped
Technical					
Laboratory	Epilepsy	50	15	42	27
	Cerebral palsy	63	63	64	40
X ray	Epilepsy	58	39	52	53
	Cerebral palsy	88	63	64	20
Physiotherapy	Epilepsy	—	—	—	—
	Cerebral palsy	75	63	36	0
Supportive					
Public health	Epilepsy	92	92	0	80
	Cerebral palsy	63	63	40	20
Psychologist or psychiatrist	Epilepsy	83	62	76	47
	Cerebral palsy	100	62	50	40
Social worker	Epilepsy	83	85	83	57
	Cerebral palsy	87	50	57	40
Vocational rehabilitation	Epilepsy	100	100	96	87
	Cerebral palsy	83	100	71	70

[a]Percentage of physicians (n = 79) reporting use "rarely" or "never"

physician, while the treatment of the disease as such, is left to the specialist. However, it was also apparent that neither the specialist nor the primary physician was addressing adequately many of the less specific but equally important nonmedical needs of these children, mainly those in the psychosocial sphere. As Table 3 indicates, when this question was explored in a birth defects clinic [9] and in an arthritis clinic [10], a majority of parents reported that neither physician had provided general advice about the care of the child on a day-to-day basis, help in making plans for the future, or genetic counseling. About one-third reported insufficient help with coordination, support, and problems related to schooling.

DISCUSSION

It is probable that the limited success of calling the attention of doctors to the consequences of dividing responsibilities in the manner described is largely attributable to economic factors arising from the manner in which most

TABLE 3. Consequences of Divided Responsibilities[a] [9] [b]

Health care area	Spina bifida (n = 44)	Rheumatoid arthritis (n = 44)	Provided by
Evaluation and treatment of the chronic disease	0	2	Specialists 100–86%
Well-child care	14	5	PMD[a] 73–70%
Acute illness care	25	9	PMD 62%
Education about the disease	9	18	Specialists 68–73%
Coordination of care	18	27	Specialists 63–55%
Support to parents	30	18	Specialists 32–59%
Genetic counseling	38	77	Specialists 42–9%
Advice about daily management	68	55	Specialists 19–43%
Planning for future	80	77	Specialists 9–11%

[a]Percentage of parents reporting services not provided by specialist or primary physician (PMD)
[b]Reprinted with permission

pediatrics is practiced in North America at present [11]. Fee for service, and even some forms of salaried employment, are not conducive to a decision to invest more time and occasionally more resources, to ensure care of the kind most of us here would advocate. Accordingly, other means must be found to help doctors practice medicine in such a manner that both the psychosocial and the more narrow medical needs are met fully and with the same degree of competence. To do so will probably require 1) modifications in education or training, 2) changes in the financial structure of health care or other types of incentives, and perhaps 3) basic alterations in the organization and delivery of health services to these children.

Educational developments alone may still succeed in producing the type of primary care practitioners described by Draper and Smits in a recent paper [12]. According to the authors, these practitioners rather than being viewed as "low level generalists" would more appropriately be thought of as "specialists whose work demands specific skills, ie as managers, advocates, educators, and counselors for their patients, as well as coordinators of other professionals involved in primary care."

The wisdom and desirability of these recommendations cannot be disputed, and perhaps in time they will come about. But we must be realistic about the likelihood that they could or would be implemented by most physicians practicing at present [13]. For doctors in the future to have the skills or inclination to accomplish these tasks will require radical alterations in both basic medical education and in training for primary care [14].

A second possibility, mentioned previously, is to place still greater emphasis for the care of these children in the hands of teams consisting of subspecialists and their colleagues, located, as a rule, in medical centers or teaching hospitals. But even with the help of such teams, each member of which is included in an attempt to meet a different area of need of either the child or his family, there is little evidence that such an approach will assuredly produce the intended results [15].

Our assessment of this approach in the 2 clinic settings described revealed many deficiencies even when the team included a pediatrician, rheumatologist, social worker, family counselor, physical therapist, and an occupational therapist! It seems that by their very nature teams diffuse rather than concentrate responsibility. The relatively scant literature on the subject suggests that frequently one member emerges as the person with whom the parent identifies most readily; not surprisingly, perhaps, it is often a physical therapist or some other member with whom frequent contact is experienced rather than the social worker or physician to whom the parent turns for advice or support in matters of health in its most broad definition.

Finally, because of the pessimism many of us share about making either of these foci of care work in the manner required, we must begin to give serious consideration to the establishment of a national network of centralized facilities specifically designed for the provision and coordination of truly comprehensive services. Over the past 2 years much of our effort in Rochester went into developing a Children's Rehabilitation Program that would undertake to remedy many of the deficiencies described. Operating on a regional basis for a population of 200,000–300,000 children, a program similar in many respects to the regional direction centers proposed in the Rand Corporation report [16] may be one answer.

Such a program, or center, ought to have the ability and staff such that each of the principal recommendations made by Brewer and Kakalik [16] could be carried out. The problems they identified are similar to those arising from our own studies: inequity in the accessibility to, and level of services from area to area and among different handicaps; gaps in services, particularly in prevention, case-finding, and direction or referral; insufficient information about the benefits or effectiveness of programs or even about who is served and who is not. As they noted, "In some programs, no one really knows who is doing what for whom or with what effect." The authors of this timely national study concluded that the service system is "varied, fragmented, uncoordinated and not particularly responsible to an individual's needs." Consequently the report calls for several major changes.

In addition to the creation of regional direction centers, the following recommendations are made with respect to medical treatment: 1) evaluation of maternal and child health programs, 2) consolidation of Medicaid and crippled children's service programs, 3) improved Medicaid program operations, 4) improved collection and use of data about medical treatment, and 5) narrowing the gap between research and medical applications. Although this report was based upon observations of services for handicapped children in the US many of the problems identified and solutions proposed, seem equally applicable to Canada, Britain, and other European countries.

CONCLUSIONS

The adequacy of medical care for children with developmental disorders has been examined from several perspectives. Based on relatively little evidence, it appears that the majority of children with major physical disorders (such as cerebral palsy or spina bifida) are detected reasonably early in most communities and thereafter receive reasonably good medical care. On the other hand, there is evidence to suggest that a majority of those with more subtle developmental disorders (such as those which affect speech or learning and minor forms of mental retardation) remain undetected.

The adequacy of care at the level of the family as a whole also needs to be scrutinized objectively. It is appropriate therefore that this session deals with the health care of both the child and the family. Innumerable studies attest to the extent to which family life can be affected by the presence of a handicapped child [17]. The force of this impact is usually the result of the physical burdens and anxieties associated with the child's care. In some cases it is also a function of some of the secondary developmental consequences of these disabilities, particularly if they affect schooling or behavior. In the Isle of Wight survey, for example, Rutter and his colleagues showed that the problems for a family with a child whose handicap was predominately behavioral were often greater than those for families with a child who had a physical disability alone [18]. It stands to reason that when both problems coexist the burden can be enormous.

Most physicians recognize, intellectually at least, the subtle interplay that occurs between the problems of the child and those of the family. They know that these forces operate in both directions: that not only may a child with a handicap impose great difficulties for his family but, as we have shown, the quality of family life may be a key determinant of the child's ability to adjust to his disorder.

However, if we understand these forces and wish to adopt a holistic approach to the family, how is this to be accomplished in our present health care system? The fact is that it is extremely rare (at least in North America) for *all* members of a family to receive care from the same physician. And in spite of much rhetoric to the contrary, the fact is that most children are cared for by doctors who know little about the basic problems, medical or otherwise, of the child's parents or sibs.

In a recently completed study [19] we found large variations between the level of knowledge of individual doctors about the families of patients they had seen the previous day. (It was only the exceptional doctor whose rudimentary knowledge of the family of any patient was at a level approaching being complete!) Furthermore there was relatively little difference between those trained as family doctors and those trained as pediatricians and almost as little difference between those who had or had not received training aimed at increasing their competence in matters relating to the family.

In summary, although some of the quantitative aspects of health care provided for children with developmental disabilities may be adequate, there is good evidence that for most such children the qualitative aspects of care are sadly deficient. And it is on these that secondary prevention is based.

It should be clear that in this paper the term "health care" has been interpreted to mean much more than "medical treatment." There may be little reason to doubt the adequacy or quality of treatment as such provided for most children with developmental disabilities. If anything there may be reason to suspect that because so many forms of therapy remain of unproven value, many children with chronic disorders may even be over treated! To cite but one example, the efficacy, let alone the effectiveness, of physical therapy for most children with cerebral palsy is still not established [20]. Within other more traditional areas of medical treatment the question of efficacy is even less clear.

Nevertheless there is probably little point in making too much of the possible limitations of many forms of therapy. In the course of providing such treatment some good may occur in other areas, and it is probable that little in the way of harm results except through the costs incurred. What is of concern, however, is the undue emphasis placed on such treatment relative to the neglect of the broader aspects of management which is equally an essential part of health care. Our task is not simply to provide the best possible technical care aimed at restoring mobility, vision, hearing, and the like, but to address with equal expertise the other needs of the child and his family [21]. On the whole the evidence suggests that we fail to do so except in isolated cases and in isolated settings. The reasons for this failure are multiple: a lack of imagination and courage in the development of programs; medical training that is narrow and unbalanced; and perhaps most importantly, the formidable barriers that derive from the way health care is organized and delivered in most Western countries.

To remedy these shortcomings is not an easy task. As knowledge increases it becomes ever more difficult for any single person, physician or otherwise, to maintain sufficient mastery of it to wish to proceed independently.

There is every reason to plead humility and defer to one's more knowledgeable colleagues. But, with increasing specialization, the child's care becomes ever more fractionated. We must ask whether in the long run the trade-off between the expert knowledge required in some areas is worth the price of removing the physician who should, theoretically, know the child and his family best from the central role that he and he alone can play.

This is the challenge involved in trying to provide truly expert and fully comprehensive health care for children with developmental disorders. It is not one that we have yet conquered, nor are we likely to do so until we face squarely the many complex issues and conflicts highlighted at this seminar.

REFERENCES

1. Pless, I. B., and Roghmann, K.: Chronic illness and its consequences: Results from three epidemiologic surveys. J. Pediatr. 79:351, 1971.
2. Rutter, M., Tizard, J., and Whitmore, K. (eds.): "Education, Health and Behavior." London: Longmans, 1970.
3. Pless, I. B., and Pinkerton, P.: "Chronic Childhood Disorder – Promoting Patterns of Adjustment." London: Kimptons, 1975, p. 31.
4. Haggerty, R. J., Roghmann, K., and Pless, I. B. (eds.): "Child Health and the Community." New York: John Wiley and Sons, 1975.
5. Pless, I. B., and Satterwhite, B.: Chronic illness. Ibid., p. 78.
6. Pless, I. B., and Satterwhite, B.: A measure of family functioning and its application. Soc. Sci. Med. 7:613, 1973.
7. Pless, I. B., and Satterwhite, B.: Chronic illness in childhood: Selection, activities and evaluation of non-professional family counsellors. Clin. Pediatr. 11:403, 1972.
8. Pless, I. B., Satterwhite, B., and VanVechten, D.: Chronic illness in childhood: A regional survey of care. Pediatrics. (In press.)

9. Kanthor, H., Pless, I. B., Satterwhite, B., and Myers, G.: Areas of responsibility in the health care of multiply handicapped children. Pediatrics 54:779, 1974.
10. Satterwhite, B., VanVechten, D., and Pless, I. B.: Divided responsibilities: Care of children with chronic disorders. (Submitted for publication.)
11. McInerny, T. K., Satterwhite, B., Sutherland, S., and Pless, I. B.: An attempt by a university Department of Pediatrics to influence the implementation of medical advances in one community. (Abstract) (Submitted to American Pediatric Society Meeting, 1976.)
12. Draper, P., and Smits, H. L.: The primary care practitioners-specialist or jack-of-all-trades. N. Engl. J. Med. 293:903, 1975.
13. Levine, M. S., Rauh, J. L., Levine, C. W., and Rubinstein, J. H.: Adolescents with developmental disabilities: A survey of their problems and their management. Clin. Pediatr. 14:25, 1975.
14. Hudson, J. I., and Nourse, E. S.: Perspectives in primary care education. J. Med. Educ. 50(12) part 2, 1975.
15. Schour, M., and Clemmens, R. L.: Fate of recommendations for children with school-related problems following interdisciplinary evaluation. J. Pediatr. 84:903, 1974.
16. Brewer, G. D., and Kakalik, J. S.: Improving services to handicapped children: Summary and analysis. Rand Corporation report R-1420/1-HEW, May 1974.
17. Pless, I. B., and Pinkerton, P.: "Chronic Childhood Disorders – Promoting Patterns of Adjustment," op. cit., pp. 163–167.
18. Rutter, M., Tizard, J., and Whitmore, K. (eds.): "Education, Health and Behavior," op. cit., pp. 330–344.
19. Vance, J. C., VanVechten, D., and Pless, I. B.: Do primary care physicians know the families they treat? (Abstract) (Submitted to Ambulatory Pediatric Association Meeting, 1976.)
20. Wright, T., and Nicholson, J.: Physiotherapy for the spastic child: An evaluation. Dev. Med. Child Neurol. 15:146, 1973.
21. Adams, M.: Social aspects of medical care for the mentally retarded. N. Engl. J. Med. 286:635, 1972.

An Interpretation of the Early Evolution of Care and Treatment of Crippled Children in the United States

Saul Benison, PhD

The deformity that marks the cripple, whether caused by accident of birth or disease, or that is the result of injury of war or work, has a strange power. On the one hand it disinherits the victim of his place in society; and on the other hand it endows him with a unique history — a history of injustice, exploitation, and ridicule. The cripple not only has to overcome his own deformity, he has also to scale the barriers that history has erected [1]. He has, for example, to overcome the vision of the cripple as seen by Peter Breughel and Hieronymous Bosch. He also has to learn to cope with the heritage of hopelessness left by the crippled and maimed who have gone before. The poet Alexander Pope's lament, "This long disease my life," is part of his heritage [2]. Lady Mary Wortley Montague's savage characterization of Pope (he was about 4 feet 6 inches high, very humpbacked and deformed)

"But as thou Pope hatst, be hated by mankind,
And with the emblem of thy crooked mind
Marked on thy back like Cain, by God's own hand,
Wander like him, accursed through the land." [p. 12, Ref. 2]

is also part of his heritage.

If we cannot forgive Richard III his villainies we might at least try to understand the development of his psychology. Shakespeare put it this way.

"I that am rudely stamped, and want love's majesty
To strut before an ambling wanton nymph;
I that am curtailed of this fair proportion,
Cheated of feature by dissembling nature,
Deformed, unfinished, sent before my time
Into this breathing world, scarce half made up,
And that so lamely and unfashionable
That dogs bark at me as I halt by them;"

These deformities, Shakespeare goes on to tell us, had an extraordinary result.

"Since I cannot prove a lover
To entertain these fair well spoken days,
I am determined to prove a villian." [3]

Richard III's psychology is also part of our cripple's heritage. Although I hasten to add that most cripples are not kings, and the singular power they generally have intimate acquaintance of is not the power of the state, but poverty.

A little more than a generation ago, Dr. Fred Albee in his autobiography expressed his view of the world of the crippled and maimed in sharp uncompromising terms: "It is not enough to pity the sick and the crippled; it is not enough to give them charity. The sick and the crippled are an economic waste. It is criminal nonsense to point to the old law of the survival of the fittest and shrug our shoulders. Society itself is sick when large numbers of its people are physically inefficient" [4]. Dr. Albee then sketched a credo to guide those physicians who cared for the crippled. "The doctor can no longer stop when he has mended the wounds in the mind and spirit; he cannot stop until he has prepared his patient to take up again a useful place in society" [4]. Dr. Albee's words reflected the experience of an orthopedic surgeon who had spent 40 years of his life fighting to rebuild men. The impact of his words on the hearts and minds of his readers has never been measured. Still his words are important because they mark (roughly, of course) the end of the first century of organized effort in the United States to dispel the darkness of the cripple's world. Further, they underline the special role of the physician in the evolution of that effort. The history of the development of care of crippled and handicapped children in the United States is in part the history of the development of orthopedic surgery and pediatrics during the 19th and early 20th centuries.

It is difficult to delineate by place and date the beginnings of orthopedic surgery as a special medical discipline in the United States. Many physicians in early 19th century America engaged in orthopedic surgery and, some like Philip Syng Physick and John Rhea Barton, were reputed to be extraordinarily skillful orthopedists. There were undoubtedly others. Yet during the first 3 decades of the last century there were no hospitals or clinics where a surgeon might devote himself exclusively to orthopedics [5, 6]. One of the first to attempt the establishment of a special orthopedic hospital in the United States was Dr. Valentine Mott — one of the most noted surgeons in New York City in the mid 19th century. In 1841, Mott proposed in the pages of *The American Journal of Medical Sciences* That, "an orthopedic institution be established at Bloomingdale for treatment of curvature of the spine and clubfeet." Mott's previous inspection of the work of European orthopedic surgeons and hospitals had convinced him that the establishment of such a hospital in the United States would be of benefit to many patients suffering from a variety of bodily deformities. Mott had the perspicacity to see the need, but few physicians responded to his call, and his plans died aborning [7]. Ironically, at approximately the same time, other physicians began to work in orthopedic surgery, and without great fanfare, ultimately accomplished what Mott wanted to do.

In 1837, Dr. William Ludwig Detmold, a graduate of the University of Gottingen, and trained in orthopedics by Louis Strohmeyer, brought Strohmeyer's tenotomy operation to New York City and began treating clubfeet and other orthopedic ailments with that technique. Detmold, a skillful surgeon, attracted many patients. By 1841, he had succeeded in establishing a public clinic for the treatment of crippled children at the College of Physicians and Surgeons in New York. He continued the clinic until 1861, when he left to serve in the Union Army during the Civil War [6, 7].

In Boston, Dr. John Ball Brown, trained in medicine by apprenticeship rather than formal schooling, turned in middle age from a successful career in general surgery to specialize in orthopedics. He adopted this new specialty because he lost a son through inflammation of the spinal cord; and he had a second son who was an invalid with lateral curvature of the spine. In 1838, Brown opened the Orthopedic Infirmary, later the Boston Orthopedic Institution, for treatment of spinal deformities and clubfeet. Brown, like Detmold, performed tenotomies. He also depended on exercise, as well as a wide variety of mechanical devices which he skillfully invented and made [8]. There were others, Dr. Louis Bauer, a graduate of the University of Berlin, established the Orthopedic Institution of Brooklyn in 1854, a year after his immigration to America. Some years later he began lecturing to students at the Brooklyn Medical and Surgical Institute. In 1864, these lectures were published in a book titled *Lectures in Orthopedic Surgery,* one of the first text books devoted to that subject in the United States [9, 10].

I don't mean to catalog the achievements of 19th century orthopedic surgeons. The lives of Detmold, Ball, and Bauer illustrate 2 important developments in orthopedic surgery — first, the rather rapid emergence of formal instruction in orthopedic surgery, and second, the tendency of many orthopedic pioneers to organize special hospitals for the treatment of crippled and deformed children. By 1861 orthopedic surgery was formally introduced into the medical curriculum of a number of medical schools. In that year, for example, Dr. Lewis Albert Sayre, a graduate of the College of Physicians and Surgeons and visiting surgeon to Bellevue Hospital, was appointed the first Professor of Orthopedic Surgery, Fractures and Dislocations at the Bellevue Hospital Medical College. For the next 32 years, Sayre not only trained generations of medical students in principles of orthopedics, he also developed special techniques for treatment of tuberculosis of the bones. Perhaps Sayre's most successful innovation was the treatment of tuberculosis of the spine with a plaster of Paris jacket [11].

Many of the orthopedic hospitals which were founded in the 1860s not only undertook the treatment of the crippled and maimed, they undertook other functions as well. Thus the Hospital for the Ruptured and Crippled in New York, founded in 1863 by Dr. James Knight, organized a brace shop, provided facilities for academic as well as religious education, and taught trades. In sum the hospital became concerned with the rehabilitation of the crippled patient [12, 13]. When Knight was succeeded by Dr. Virgil Gibney in 1887, the hospital also became a training ground for orthopedists. When Gibney retired in 1924, he had trained 134 house officers. Of these, 9 became professors of orthopedic surgery, 18 served as assistant professors, and 18 were instructors [14, 15].

I do not mean to suggest by the foregoing achievements that all pioneer orthopedists were great or even admirable men. As a matter of fact, some of the battles between Bauer and Sayre, or Knight and Gibney, or between Russell Hibbs and Newton Shaffer [16, 17], over operating techniques or merely administrative procedures make current academic fights seem like girl scout taffy pulls. I do say that these pioneers, the institutions they founded, and the young cadres they trained, provided a fulcrum for the development of the care of the crippled and handicapped in the 20th century. But they were not alone.

The development of pediatrics in the United States in a measure parallels the evolution of orthopedic surgery. While the immediate concerns of pediatrics were not mending and rehabilitating the handicapped, pediatrics nevertheless also played a singular role in the evolution of the treatment and care of the crippled. Its importance stems from its contributions to preventive medicine, and more especially, its role in fostering a social environment conducive to the optimum growth of children.

During the first three quarters of the 19th century, there were few physicians in the United States who devoted themselves exclusively to the treatment of children's diseases. While it is true that one can cite the names of notable 19th and early 20th century pediatricians such as Abraham Jacobi, Job Lewis Smith, Joseph O'Dwyer, Henry Koplik, Thomas Rotch and others, pediatrics as a medical specialty developed very slowly. For example, although the first hospitals devoted exclusively to diseases of children were organized as early as 1854 and 1855, the children's hospital movement essentially remained moribund until the late 1870s and 1880s. Indeed, by 1892, there were only 29 children's hospitals in the U.S., and the majority of these were concentrated in such large urban centers as New York, Philadelphia, Boston, Chicago, and San Francisco. The first medical journal devoted exclusively to pediatric problems only appeared in 1884, and it wasn't until 1888 that a National Pediatric Society was founded. Local pediatric societies did not appear before the mid 1890s [18].

The physician whose career perhaps best epitomizes the growth of pediatrics in the United States at the end of the 19th century was Dr. Luther Emmet Holt. In a measure Holt's interest in diseases of children can be traced to his experience as a student intern at the Hospital of the Ruptured and Crippled in New York. It is known, for example, that it was Holt's exposure to the problems of crippled children that led to his graduation dissertation on *Articular Osteitis of the Hip Joint.* Following the receipt of his MD degree from the College of Physicians and Surgeons in New York in 1880, and an internship at Bellevue, Holt undertook special pediatric studies in Europe. In 1889, after several years of training in various children's hospitals in New York, Holt was appointed physician-in-chief to the then newly founded Babies Hospital. Two years later he was called to be Professor of Pediatrics at the New York Polyclinic Hospital and Medical School.

It is difficult to say where Holt made his mark first, whether at the child's bedside as a clinician, or as a teacher. In either case it was the sick child who was his concern. His textbooks on *The Care and Feeding of Children* and *Diseases of Infancy and Childhood,* taught generations of physicians and nurses. Indeed, the Babies Hospital became the training ground for both nurses and physicians interested in childhood diseases, and more especially the scientific investigation of problems of infant metabolism and infant nutrition [19].

One facet of Holt's work which perhaps best mirrors the impact of pediatric thought and practice in preventive medicine and ultimately the care of the crippled, was working out standards of clean milk production. In this work Holt was at one with other pediatric pioneers, such as Dr. Daniel Coit of Newark, New Jersey, and Dr. Thomas Rotch of Harvard, who helped organize the certified milk movement in the United States [20–23]. The clean milk campaign was one of several campaigns that pediatricians engaged in during the first decade of the 20th century to cut down infant mortality [24]. Perhaps the best index of the growth of this concern was the establishment of the Bureau of Child Hygiene in the New York City Department of Health in 1908 and the United States Children's Bureau in 1913. Both of these agencies helped foster an environment of health and in a deep sense are a monument to the growth of pediatric thought [25, 26]. The end of Dr. Holt's career mirrored these new concerns of pediatricians. In the last 4 years of his life, Holt devoted himself to the Child Health Organization, an agency which was formed after World War I to educate a new generation of children in health practice. Its ultimate goal was to prevent in the future the deplorable physical state of the draftees of World War I [19].

I don't want to suggest that pediatricians as a body threw themselves into health preservation campaigns without question. When Dr. Thomas Rotch in 1909 called on members of the American Pediatric Society to take an active role in the solution of social problems affecting the health and welfare of children, he was roundly attacked by such distinguished pediatricians as Dr. Isaac Abt of Chicago on the grounds that it was not the purpose of the Society to become entangled in political or legislative questions [27]. Five years later, Dr. Sam Hammill in a Presidential address to the same Society, proclaimed that preventive medicine required the pediatrician to take an active role in all public health questions. Indeed Dr. Hammill was of the conviction that pediatricians should preempt the field, and he looked upon social workers and philanthropists who worked in this area as a burden [28]. Yet even as Dr. Hammill spoke, it was too late for the pediatrician to play an exclusive role, and more especially in the care and treatment of crippled children. By the beginning of the 20th century, the crippled child was no longer simply a medical problem. The dramatic increase of such crippling diseases as polio, TB, and rickets, as well as the disabling effects of child labor, had transformed him into a social problem. As such he became the concern not only of social workers and philanthropists but of state and federal legislators as well [29, 30].

It is a matter of some moment that the earliest expression of governmental concern with the care and treatment of crippled children did not occur on a national level, but rather on a state level. In 1896, Dr. Arthur Gillette, a young orthopedic surgeon, presented a paper to a Minnesota Conference on Charities and Corrections with the then novel thesis that the state had the obligation to erect a state hospital for the care and treatment of crippled children. Gillette's paper gained state-wide attention, and the following year when he made a similar proposal to the state legislature, the legislature authorized the State Board of Regents to provide for treatment and care of indigent crippled children in hospitals within 10 miles of the state university. To carry out the act, the state provided $5,000 a year for the next 2 years [31]. At best it was a modest beginning but it was a beginning. Two years later, Dr. Newton Shaffer, Professor of Orthopedic Surgery at Cornell, with the approval of Governor Theodore Roosevelt, introduced a similar bill in the New York State legislature. In April of 1900, the legislature authorized $15,000 for the erection and maintenance of "a hospital for indigent crippled and deformed children." The hospital, originally conceived of as a convalescent hospital, had 25 beds. Within a year there were over 500 applications for a place in the hospital [32, 33].

In 1899, Dr. Lenore Perky, a young physician, moved by the pathetic condition of the indigent crippled children she discovered in the appropriately named Nebraska House for the Friendless, began a campaign among physicians and legislators to provide for state care and treatment of such unfortunates. Initially she was rebuffed by both physicians and legislators. In 1905, after 6 years of agitation she persuaded the legislature to establish a state hospital for the care of indigent ruptured and crippled children of Nebraska. Of all the early legislative efforts to establish a state hospital for the indigent crippled, Nebraska proved the most difficult to accomplish. The original bill, which called for an appropriation of $25,000, was cut to $10,000. The governor initially refused to sign the amended bill on the grounds there were not enough crippled in Nebraska to people the hospital. Only when it was demonstrated that there were many more cripples in the state capital alone than the governor required, did he sign the bill. Still, despite its difficult beginning the hospital established by the Nebraska legislature proved the most successful of all state hospitals for crippled children and remained a model for other states in the years that followed [34, 35]. In part, its success was the result of excellent staffing. The original superintendent and his assistant, Dr. John Lord and Dr. Winnett Orr were well trained and skillful surgeons. Their superintendent of nurses, Mary Hardwicke, was trained at the Hospital for the Ruptured and Crippled by Dr. Virgil Gibney and Dr. Royal Whitman. With Miss Hardwicke's cooperation a training school for orthopedic nurses was started at the hospital [34, 35]. Most important of all, the hospital from the beginning conceived its function not only to treat and care for patients, but to educated and rehabilitate them as well.

In 1916, Dr. Orr summarized the achievements of Nebraska State Hospital during its first decade as follows: "Almost daily we are asked to express in figures different phases of our work. We can tell for example, that care of our patients is costing the State of Nebraska about 30¢ per day for food, 60¢ per day for hospital care, and 15½¢ per day for schooling... Also people are always interested to know that during the ten years of this hospital's existence we have expended nearly $100,000 on our plant and that the actual care and education of the 1,200 patients received during that time has involved an outlay of about $250,000, or in round figures, about $200 per patient. On the same basis we find that our patients for the entire period have remained at the hospital on an average of about 180 days... Also during this period more than 1,000 operations have been done. Many thousands of plaster casts and braces have been put on and hundreds of greatly benefited and cured patients have been discharged from the institution. To use figures again, approximately 750 to 800 of all the patients treated at the hospital have been discharged as cured or substantially improved" [35, pp. 24, 25].

Not all states acted in as generous a fashion as New York, Minneota, or Nebraska. Before World War I only 5 states established state hospitals for the care, treatment and education of the indigent crippled. The 32 other hospitals that existed were in the main supported by private philanthropic funds. The reaction of some states when asked for such help would have made Scrooge appear saintly. From 1906 to 1918 the State of New Hampshire was asked to make an annual appropriation of $1,000 for the orthopedic care of the indigent crippled. Each year the legislature refused. In 1919 it finally relented and made an appropriation of $2,500 [36]. In other states private benefactors assumed burdens that might well have been shouldered by the state. Following the polio epidemic of 1914 in Vermont, Redfield Proctor made an anonymous grant to Dr. Robert Lovett of Boston to hold public clinics for polio victims. Lovett, with the assistance of his nurse Wilhelmina Wright, held such clinics, in 5 different state centers. It was during the course of these clinics that Lovett, in collaboration with Dr. Earl Martin, developed quantitative tests to evaluate the muscle strength of crippled polio victims. Later Mr. Proctor and his sister helped establish Ormsbee House, a convalescent hospital for polio victims, near Proctor, Vermont [37].

The care of the crippled varied from state to state, and no state proved to be free of problems. In 1919, for example, 46 Rotary Clubs in Ohio constituted themselves into an organization called The Ohio Society for Crippled Children and submitted a plan to the state legislature that modified ongoing techniques of providing medical and surgical treatment for indigent crippled children. Under this new plan the State Board of Charities, upon receiving notice that there were parents who were unwilling or unable to provide treatment for their crippled children, could, after consultation with the Court, arrange to take custody of such children, and put them in a hospital which in their judgment could provide the necessary treatment. If parents could not pay the costs of necessary treatment and education, the State Board of Charities would assume the burden of such costs out of their own funds [38, 39].

The modifications suggested by The Ohio Plan was one indication of the shortcomings of some existing state care plans for crippled children. An investigation by a special commission of the New York State Legislature in 1924 turned up others. The investigators here discovered that while there appeared to be enough beds in state hospitals for acute cases of crippling, there were not enough beds for convalescents. Equally bad, there was no adequate provision for schooling long-term crippled convalescents. Perhaps the most serious criticism the investigating committee made was that no one assumed any responsibility for the crippled preschool child, although more than 50% of all crippling conditions occurred in children of this age group [40].

The administration of hospitals for the crippled was not the only problem which absorbed those who cared for and treated crippled children at the turn of the century. Education of such children was another even more pressing problem. There had been guide markers for the solution of such problems before 1900. For example, the Hospital for the Ruptured and Crippled in New York, had from its inception in 1863 wisely provided for both a regular and vocational education program [41]. But few institutions followed its example; most simply designed programs to acclimate crippled children to living in the hospital and little more.

One of the first physicians to address himself to the educational needs of the crippled was Dr. Edward H. Bradford, Professor of Orthopedic Surgery at Harvard. In 1893, Bradford with the help of a friend, Dr. Augustus Thorndike, founded The Industrial School for Crippled and Deformed Children in Boston [42, 43]. Bradford, in the words of a contemporary, Louise Eberle, "had the singular perception that if cripples could be educated as a matter of charity, they could also be educated for taking them out of the charity class" [44]. It is difficult to say whether Bradford's vision was in fact singular, or whether he was the first to establish such a school. What is important is that the idea seemed to be in the air. In 1890, the Rhinelander sisters in New York City erected a building on East 80th Street in Manhattan so that The Children's Aid Society could provide a grade school and vocational training program for crippled children [45]. In 1900, the Association for the Aid of Crippled Children, in concert with the Emanuel Lehman Foundation, opened The Crippled Children's East Side Free School on

Henry Street "to improve the children's physical condition, to train them to become self-supporting and to provide them with work" [46]. Such schools quickly proliferated through the country. In 1906, P. A. B. Widener of Philadelphia opened The Widener Memorial School for Crippled Children as a memorial to his wife and eldest son, perhaps the most well endowed and lavish hospital school in the country [47]. There were other such hospitals as well as other educational programs. In 1910, led by The Association for the Aid of Crippled Children in New York, efforts were made to introduce classes for crippled children in urban schools. This program also caught on, and soon, Boards of Education in various urban centers introduced similar classes into regular schools or else set aside special schools for those crippled who could leave their homes [48]. Philanthropists and educators, one might say, had in concert taken the first steps for the rehabilitation of the crippled and handicapped.

There was, however, one problem with all of these educational programs. They were too special. They all focused exclusively on the crippled; no one thought it necessary to educate the so-called "normal" members of the population to the problems of the crippled.

As early as the 1890s, various charity organization societies established special bureaus to obtain employment for the handicapped. Invariably these bureaus failed, not because there wasn't enough work that cripples might do. They failed because no one wanted to employ cripples. In 1908, the Social Research Committee of the Russell Sage Foundation, in cooperation with the Bureau of the Handicapped of the New York Charity Organization, investigated existing employment opportunities for the handicapped and disabled. They soon discovered that while there were many jobs which were available, few cripples were hired because they lacked the necessary skills required to work effectively. Ironically the Bureau eventually had to close its doors because it lacked facilities to provide the skilled training it earlier reported was needed. In 1914, rehabilitation workers, led by *The American Journal of Care for Cripples,* began to agitate for special programs to educate the handicapped to a wider spectrum of vocational opportunities than those traditionally provided for by caning, embroidery or jewelry making [49].

There can be no doubt that the need for vocational rehabilitation existed long before World War I. Living and working in an industrial society created far many more cripples and handicapped than the epidemic of trauma that is called war. Still all efforts to obtain federal assistance for a national vocational education bill before World War I failed — except in one instance. In 1917, Congress established a Board for Vocational Education whose purpose was to supervise the federal funds granted to aid existing state vocational education programs [49].

It has been argued in some quarters that war ultimately leads to some good. Some historians have even justified the carnage of the American Civil War on the grounds that it provided the first 4-year program devoted to medicine and surgery in the United States. If Congress, before 1918, could avoid facing the problems of the worker who was crippled in the daily industrial war, it could not easily avoid dealing with the problems of rehabilitating disabled soldiers and sailors. Although I must add that it tried. In 1920, after almost 2 years of debate and consultation with physicians, government agencies, and social workers, Congress passed a law which in essence provided federal aid to such states as would provide matching funds for the vocational rehabilitation of disabled soldiers and sailors. Such rehabilitation for civilians was not provided for until several years later. There was no lack of willingness on the part of physicians and social workers to instruct the Congress on the meaning of vocational rehabilitation; the difficulty was in getting it to listen. Fortunately, however, there proved to be less difficulty in getting the various state legislatures to listen [49].

One of the most successful state rehabilitation programs was that begun by New Jersey. The philosophy that guided it was that of Dr. Fred Albee. "By rehabilitation," he later wrote, "is not meant only the latest methods of orthopedic surgery and surgical reconstruction of the injured, but also training of the injured member to perform the utmost function of which it is capable. The teaching of the patient skill in work other than that which he has been doing... The application of the latest psychological methods to improve his morale and finally a study of industry for the purpose of ascertaining those occupations which are suited to the cripple" [50]. For Albee the work in rehabilitation fell into 3 main categories:

"1st Physical reconstruction — that is repair of the injury — which depends on the medical profession
2nd Vocational rehabilitation — which depends on education
3rd Job restoration — which depends on industry" [50].

Albee's vision of rehabilitation was much better than that of the Congress. His rehabilitation plan was not only to care for disabled soldiers and sailors, but for workers injured in industry, as well as those crippled by disease, or born with congenital malformations. Albee's plans and subsequent achievements for the New Jersey Rehabilitation Commission shines as a bright light in the early history of the care and treatment of the crippled in the United States [50].

There were, however, other programs which proved just as valuable. Not the least of these was the construction of special hospitals for the care and treatment of the crippled by Masons, Shriners, Elks, and Rotarians [51, 52], as well as the extraordinary International Society for Crippled Children, which propagandized endlessly on behalf of the crippled child and his rights throughout the 1920s and 1930s [53]. There was also darkness — especially that created by a federal government which would not easily accept its responsibilities to care for the nation's stated ideals "of providing for the general welfare."

EPILOGUE

Following the passage of the Federal Rehabilitation Act of 1920, Congress did little to help the crippled in the United States, unless one considers the various amendments offered to the original act during the debates on new appropriations. These amendments, however, changed little of substance in the original Act [54]. Actually the only federal agency to concern itself with the care and treatment of crippled children during the 1920s was the Children's Bureau. In 1924, Dr. Edwards A. Park of the Pediatric Department of the Yale Medical School and Dr. Martha Eliot working under the mandate of the Children's Bureau "to investigate the diseases of children," undertook a study of the prevention and cure of rickets, then one of the major crippling diseases of children in the United States. In 1925, the Bureau followed this seminal study with an investigation of the provisions of various state laws for the care and treatment of crippled children, covering such subjects as techniques for locating and diagnosing crippled children, hospital and convalescent care, education, and last, but certainly not least, the status and the effectiveness of private agencies caring for crippled children. While these studies had no immediate political impact, they nevertheless proved extraordinarily useful. A decade later they helped educate the legislators drawing up the Social Security Act [55].

The Social Security Act of 1935 marked a turning point in the concern of the federal government in the care and treatment of crippled children. Under Title Five of that Act, the Children's Bureau was charged with administering federal aid to states for various maternal and children's care programs, including crippled children. Although the aid was ultimately administered by an agency designated by the state, (usually the State Health Department or State Department of Education) no funds were forthcoming from the Bureau until the state held a census of crippled children and came up with a program for their care and treatment. By the end of 1938, 47 state plans of services for crippled children were approved and in operation [55].

While there is no gainsaying the importance of federal programs under the New Deal in focusing national attention on the needs of crippled children, an equally important impetus to the development of the care and treatment of such children came from programs of private foundations, especially those sponsored by The National Foundation—March of Dimes in Professional Education. Beginning in 1939, these programs included setting up training and treatment centers for polio, instituting teaching programs in medical schools in physical medicine and rehabilitation, and above all providing grants to various schools for the training of orthopedic nurses, physiotherapists, and social workers. In so doing, The National Foundation accomplished what the government had neglected. In sum, The

Foundation helped train a cadre of professional medical workers that was to play a unique and substantive role in the subsequent development of the care and rehabilitation of the crippled in the United States.

REFERENCES

1. McMurtrie, D.: "The Disabled Soldier." New York: Macmillan Co., 1919, pp. 1–17.
2. Nicholson, M. and Rosseau, G. S.: This long disease my life. In "Alexander Pope and the Sciences." Princeton: Princeton University Press, 1968, pp. 7–82.
3. Shakespeare, W.: Richard III. Act 1, Scene 1.
4. Albee, F.H.: "A Surgeon's Fight to Rebuild Men." New York: Dutton, 1943, p. 22.
5. Shands, A. R., Jr.: "The Early Orthopedic Surgeons of America." St. Louis: C. V' Mosby Co., 1970.
6. Keith, A. (ed.): "Menders of the Maimed." London: Oxford Medical Publications, 1919, pp. 173–175.
7. Shands, A. R., Jr.: op. cit., pp. 2–15.
8. Ibid., pp. 128–133.
9. Ibid., pp. 16–19.
10. Keith, A., op. cit., pp. 175–177.
11. Shands, A. R., Jr., op. cit., pp. 30–49.
12. Ibid., pp. 69–84.
13. Bick, E. M.: "Source Book of Orthopedics." New York: Hafner, 1968, p. 492.
14. Ibid., p. 175.
15. Shands, A. R., Jr., op. cit., pp. 85–96.
16. Ibid., pp. 24–27, p. 75, p. 19.
17. Goodwin, G. M.: "Russell L. Hibbs." New York: Columbia University Press, 1935, pp. 11–16.
18. Garrison, F. H. and Abt, A. F.: "History of Pediatrics." Philadelphia: W. B. Saunders Co., 1965, pp. 105–112; 121–124.
19. Park, E. A. and Mason, H. H. (eds.): Luther Emmet Holt. In Veeder, B. S. (ed.): "Pediatric Profiles." St. Louis: C. V. Mosby Co., 1957, pp. 30–60.
20. Talbot, F. B. and Rotch, T. M.: Ibid., 29–32.
21. Garrison, F. H. and Abt, A. F.: op. cit., pp. 141–142.
22. Coit, H. L.: "A Plan to Procure Cow's Milk Designed for Clinical Purposes," Newark, N.J., 1893.
23. Straus, L. G.: The remedy pasteurization: The life and work of Nathan Straus, New York, 1917. In Bremner, R. H. (ed.): "Children and Youth in America, A Documentary History, 1866–1932." Cambridge: Harvard University Press, vol. II, parts 7–8, pp. 867–871.
24. Ibid., pp. 875–894.
25. Baker, J. S.: "Fighting for Life." New York, 1939.
26. Bradbury, D. E.: "Five Decades of Action for Children." Washington, D. C.: Government Printing Office, 1962.
27. Rotch, T. M.: The position and work of the American Pediatric Society towards public questions, Trans. of American Pediatric Scoeity, XXI (1909). In Bremner, R. H. op. cit., pp. 821–828.
28. Hammill, S. McC.: Responsibility of the pediatrist towards the problem of public health, Trans. of American Pediatric Society, XXVI (1914). Ibid, pp. 828–831.
29. Trattner, W. L.: "Crusade for the Children." Chicago: Quadrangel Books, 1970, pp. 21–66.

30. Abt, H. E.: "The Care, Cure and Education of the Crippled Child." New York: Arno Press, 1974, pp. 12–15.
31. Ibid., p. 29.
32. Shands, A. R., Jr., op. cit., p. 117.
33. Works Progress Administration. "A Brief History of the Nebraska Orthopedic Hospital," (N.D.) (Nebraska Historical Society) p. 2.
34. Lord, J. P. and Orr, W. H.: The Nebraska State Hospital for Crippled, Ruptured and Deformed Children: The institution, its origin, development and needs. Nebraska Med. J. 1, 1907.
35. Works Progress Administration, op. cit., pp. 1–25.
36. Abt, H. E., op. cit., pp. 32–33.
37. State Department of Public Health, Vermont, "Infantile Paralysis in Vermont 1894–1922," Burlington, Vermont, 1924, pp. 201–207; 232–239; 275–288.
38. Bremner, R. H. op. cit., pp. 1033–1035.
39. Abt, H. C., op. cit., pp. 30–31.
40. New York State. "Report of the New York State Commission for Survey of Crippled Children," Document 100 (Legislative Documents Albany, 1925), cited in Bremner, R. H. op. cit., pp. 1035–1038.
41. Shands, A. R., Jr., op. cit., pp. 72–74.
42. Ibid., pp. 142–144.
43. Reeves, E.: "Care and Education of Crippled Children in the United States." New York: Arno Press, pp. 226–227.
44. Eberle, L.: "The Maimed, the Halt and the Race." Hospital Social Service VI, 1922. In Bremner, R. H., op. cit., p. 1026.
45. Reeves, E., op. cit., p. 231.
46. Ibid., pp. 228–230.
47. Ibid., pp. 173–183.
48. Ibid., pp. 56–59.
49. MacDonald, M. E.: "Federal Grants for Rehabilitation." Chicago: University of Chicago Press, 1944, pp. 7–14.
50. Alber, F. H., op. cit., pp. 219–246.
51. Bremner, R. H., op. cit., pp. 1028–1030.
52. Abt, H. E. (ed.), op. cit., pp. 19–23.
53. Ibid., pp. 205–207.
54. MacDonald, M. E., op. cit., pp. 66–70.
55. Bradbury, D. E., op. cit., pp. 26–27; 38–39; 46–48.

IV
SOCIETAL REACTION:
THE HANDICAPPED INTEGRATED INTO SOCIETY

IV

Education, Recreation, and Vocational Training

Edmund W. Gordon, Ed.D.

Efforts at providing systematic programs of education and vocational training for persons with developmental disabilities can be traced to the latter half of the 19th century. Prior to that time we find isolated efforts at the habilitation of handicapped individuals but little organized societal effort directed at the provision of such opportunities for large numbers of handicapped people. It was not until the 20th century, however, that public and private institutions began to organize habilitation and rehabilitation services which could be clearly distinguished from custodial care or at best programs of activity primarily designed to keep busy the hands of the unfortunate, lest those idle hands drift into autoerotic behaviors. It is only within the past 25 years that organized efforts have emerged to address the recreational needs of people with developmental disorders. But let me hasten to remind you that while there has been considerable time, effort, and money directed at developing systematic educational and vocational training opportunities, we as a society have been woefully remiss in directing such attention to the recreational needs of handicapped people. This neglect may be in part due to the fact that we have been able to retain a large measure of public service responsibility for education while recreational opportunities are more greatly controlled by profit-dominated free enterprise.

It is not the differential attention given to these service needs of handicapped people, however, that I want to discuss in this paper. Rather I am concerned here with an aspect of the technology which underlies all of these services and which in the long run could be more frustrating to their adequate development than are the socioeconomic structures through which these services are now provided.

The planning, design, and delivery of human services must be based upon the characteristics of the persons to be served. It is out of concern for this postulate that assessment and classification systems have been developed. In response to a perceived scarcity in the resources available for education around the end of the 19th century, Binet was given the task of developing an instrument which could be used to identify those persons whose intellectual characteristics made them most likely to benefit from the educational services then available. His test of human intelligence and the many variations of the theme which have followed were designed to assess status characteristics and provide the basis for the prediction of academic performance in ways which influenced the assignment of individuals and groups for educational services. Subsequent variations which focused on aptitudes and specific achievement in academic and vocational areas came to be used not only to assign people in relation to services to be received but also in relation to developmental and work opportunities.

This was a logical development of the time. The history of the development of Western societies has been marked by a progressively more democratic approach to the distribution of developmental opportunities. In earlier periods opportunities for education were made available to the political and religious nobility and a few lowborn persons who were lucky enough to incur their favor. Following the Protestant Reformation, political revolutions in North America and France, and the emergence of the industrial revolution, broader categories of persons were deemed to be educable and likely to benefit from education. Slowly meritocratic *class* biases replaced aristocratic *caste* biases as the basis for assignment to educational or work opportunities. It was to determine who *merited* the investment in education that intelligence and achievement testing emerged, and this implicit purpose has dominated our work in educational and vocational assessment.

Now this concern with determining who is likely to benefit from an intervention is not inappropriate; however, the heavy dependence on prediction of likely response based on measured *status* rather than analyzed *function* presents the problem. Our preoccupation in the assessment of human characteristics with the sampling of achieved status as a basis for prediction is based on the assumption that achievement at one stage of development under fairly standard conditions of learning will be repeated in subsequent stages under comparable conditions of learning. Again the position is a logical one, but knowledge and circumstances have outdistanced our technology of assessment. We now have a better knowledge base in support of Binet's ignored assertion that intelligence consists of several aspects of function, some of which may be capable of improvement with training. We now know that what surfaces as achievement is a composite of behavioral functions and that the elements which go to make up this composite vary from individual to individual and probably from situation to situation. We now know that mental functions and achievement involve both the affective and cognitive processes which interact to partially determine the quality of achievement. We now understand that current status with respect to a human characteristic is only reliable as a prediction of future achievement status if we know the developmental circumstances out of which the future achievement must arise. Put more simply, standardized tests are good predictors as long as the situation into which the subject is expected to continue learning is very much like the prior learning situation and similar to the learning situation to which the norming group has been exposed. When the learning situation is radically changed the power of our prediction is reduced.

I have suggested that it is not only the knowledge base which has changed but also the circumstances. When the assessment of achieved status came to dominate educational planning, meritocratic concepts of opportunity also dominated in our society. The 20th century, and certainly its latter half, has increasingly been marked by a shift to more democratic concepts of opportunity. Today we are able to assert a right to a thorough and adequate education as a universal right of citizenship. The walls of biased exclusion based on sex, ethnicity, class, and even on handicapped status have been shattered, and it is the rabble from their defending forces that we are now stumbling over. Not yet defeated but heavily under attack are the walls of bias based on achieved status or merit. Here, coupled with our awareness of the availability of resources adequate to guarantee thorough and adequate development for all our citizens, the question increasingly asked of educational planners and assessment specialists is not which of us are more likely to succeed but what is required of the intervention process to ensure (or at least more greatly enhance the chance of) success for each of us.

Now, when the question for education or any human service is posed in that frame, the task posed for the technology is quite different. If we are to adequately plan and deliver education, vocational training, or recreational services for any or all segments of a population as varied as is ours and if the goal is to ensure success against whatever criterion we set, the first and most urgent task is to develop a technology of assessment that is capable of producing the kind of information concerning the characteristics of those to be served that is essential to the design of the program of human service. That assessment information will include data referable to achievement status, but it must also include data which are referable to the functional characteristics of the learner. For purposes of educational planning and design it may not help much to have an intelligence or achievement quotient (a score). What is more important is information concerning the nature of the learner's behavioral function — how does she go about solving problems? What information or skill strengths or weaknesses are available to work with and under what circumstances is the learner enabled to use them in learning? What are the stylistic features of the behavior? What are the prepared response tendencies? What turns him on? Assessment data of this type are not usually made available in the process of measuring status. Yet as we look at the diverse patterns of behavior and background that children bring to school and as we observe the extent to which children's interests, energies, and abilities are wasted in our schools, it begins to be clear that schooling for all children may need to be more closely tailored to those variations in their functional characteristics which have relevance for learning.

We are particularly concerned with children who have developmental disabilities. These are children, who, in addition to such diverse characteristics as may be observed in the general population, are handicapped by conditions which may especially limit their adaptive capacities. If we have established that the normal range of variance in learner characteristics requires that we become more sensitive to functional differences in what they bring to the learning situation, it is even more essential that this approach come to dominate the technology of assessment and educational intervention for handicapped learners.

In his introduction to a little book by Else Haeussermann, *Developmental Potential of Preschool Children,* which has received too little attention, the late Herbert Birch in 1958 suggested that "the use of a method for intellectual evaluation as an instrument that has positive value for the promotion of training and education is an essential feature of rehabilitation. . . . In this area of work, one is far less concerned with predicing whether a given child will achieve success in competition with a group of age mates drawn from the general population, than with the problem of determining the kinds of training and experience that will best promote his own adaptive functional abilities." Ms. Haeussermann goes on to spell out a manual for the qualitative assessment of the functional characteristics of handicapped learners. Early in the book, as in her professional practice, she made it abundantly clear that "the purpose of the educational evaluation is to provide a basis for planning the educational program by giving the teacher systematic and detailed information about each child." The assessment processes as described and utilized by Haeussermann did not ignore the measurement of status. In areas of function which are essential to further learning, she was careful to document the developmental level at which the child functioned and indeed attempted to estimate overall developmental age for her examinees. However, this work persistently went beyond the quantitative representation of developmental level to a concern with the detailed description of the nature of adaptive function in the child's behavior. To generate these data the examination was as much an exercise in instruction as in assessment. The examiner's behavior can best be described as mieutic, ie having the character of midwifery, where the task is to aid the examinee in producing whatever adaptive functions of which he is capable. The concern is not so much can he do it under standard stimulus conditions but what are the stimulus conditions necessary to the elicitation of an appropriate response. Thus it is not only the functional characteristics of the child but also the functional characteristics of the environment which are conducive or necessary to the child's performance.

The work I refer to was published almost 20 years ago. In several clinical settings around the country aspects of this work or similar approaches have been developed and are in varying stages of implementation. But if one examines the current state of the art as practiced in public schools, in training centers for handicapped persons, or even the current state of the published technology, we find that were Ms. Haeussermann with us today, doing what she was doing 20 years ago, she would still be years ahead of contemporary practice. The psychometric industry has not adopted her approach to assessment and developed instrumentation for its implementation. We have not taught our teacher either how to conduct such evaluations or to use such evaluation data. We have not even encouraged the parents of these children to demand it. Good clinical psychologists approach the Haeussermann model in some of their efforts at differential diagnosis and testing the limits, but intensive qualitative analyses which inform the instructional process are not the routine products of their work. In the emerging field of individually prescribed instruction, we are beginning to have movement in this direction, but most of this work remains tied to relatively static measures of learning rate, or interest, or personality type.

We can explore possibilities for adding to the quantitative reports on the performance of students, reports descriptive of the patterns of achievement and function derived from the qualitative analysis of existing tests. The existing instruments should be examined with a view to categorization, factorial analysis, and interpretation to determine whether or not the data of these instruments can be reported in descriptive and qualitative ways, in addition to the traditional quantitative report.

For example, response patterns might be reported differentially for information recall (rote recall, associative recall, derivative recall) or vocabulary (absolute, contextual).

We can explore the development of test items and procedures that lend themselves to descriptive and qualitative analyses of cognitive and affective adaptive functions, in addition to a wider variety of specific achievements.

In the development of new tests, attention should be given to the appraisal of adaptation in new learning situations; problem solving in situations that require varied cognitive skills and styles; analysis, search, and synthesis behaviors; information management, processing, and utilization skills; and nonstandard information pools.

In the development of new procedures, attention should be given to the appraisal of comprehension through experiencing, listening, and looking, as well as reading; expression through artistic, oral, nonverbal, and graphic, as well as written symbolization; characteristics of temperament; sources and status of motivation; and habits of work and task involvement under varying conditions of demand.

In the development of tests and procedures designed to get at specific achievements, attention should be given to broadening the varieties of subject matter, competencies, and skills assessed; examining these achievements in a variety of contexts; open-ended and unstructured probes of achievement to allow for atypical patterns and varieties of achievement; and to assessing nonacademic achievements such as social competence, social coping skills, avocational skills, and artistic, athletic, political, or mechanical skills in nature as well as in contrived settings.

We can explore the development of report procedures that convey the qualitative richness of these new tests and procedures to students and institutions in ways that encourage individualized prescriptive educational planning. What is called for is a statement about the nature of adaptive function in each individual that lends itself to planning a way of intervening in and facilitating his development. Patterns of strength and weakness, conditions conducive to successful coping, conditions resulting in congruence and engagement or incongruence and alienation are examples of the kind of information required.

We can explore the development of research that will add to understanding of the ways in which more traditional patterns of instruction will need to be modified to make appropriate use of wider ranges and varieties of human talent and adaptation in continuing education. It would be relatively useless to identify broader ranges of behavior if these did not have their representation in programs of instruction and if opportunities for the use of these adaptive patterns in learning were not available to young people. Alongside modification of instruments of assessment and of procedures for appraisal there needs to be a considerable amount of attention given to modifying the curriculum and conditions under which teaching and learning occur.

Unfortunately not much of this thinking is reflected in the educational programs available to handicapped persons. Nor is this diagnostic, prescriptive approach to education routinely available to the general population.

Why is there this great lag in the technology of education? Pedagogic practice, as it is represented in mass education, has been influenced by the same normative bias that has dominated assessment practice. We as a profession have looked to mean and modal conditions and characteristics as the basis for the design of our educational programs. Norm-based designs are cheaper than customized approaches and for a lot of our children mass education seems to work. That is, those programs and strategies we have developed based on what most people seem to want and respond to seems to have enabled the US society to train more of its people than any other country in the history of man. We have manned our commerce and industry with a larger number of relatively skilled people than other countries. We have credentialed more of our citizens. We send more people on to higher education. For a lot of us this faulty system of education works. But for too many of us it has not worked. For blacks, Chicanos, native Americans, Puerto Ricans, many poverty-stricken whites, the mentally handicapped, the emotionally disturbed, for many people with other handicaps we have not done so well. But these people who are socially or developmentally handicapped are also the powerless members of our society, and it is always the powerless who are abused, neglected, and exploited.

The technology of education lags because its refined development has not yet been determined to be essential to the progress and survival of the nation. We are no longer able to absorb or hide our handicapped and underdeveloped people as we once were, but we are still able to ignore them. It may only be when they gain political power or are at least perceived as being essential to the nation's survival that the society will require that education refine its technology in their service.

In the presence of such a circumstance there is another alternative. Societies change by virtue of powerful political processes. They also change as the result of strong moral and intellectual forces. The intellectual and professional communities can be such a force. When, through our research and theoretical work, we inform public policy and in addition create public awareness of the potential for a higher order of human organization and service, we set the stage for the operation of moral and intellectual forces to which the nation sometimes responds. In our developmental services to handicapped people we have sometimes released such forces but not consistently so. Sometimes in our efforts at doing so we have misinformed public policy by our mistaken views of the nature of the problem with which we are dealing. Let us return for a moment to the education of handicapped people. It is only in recent years that we have begun to talk about and organize around the problems of handicapped children rather than the mentally retarded, the physically handicapped, the brain injured, etc. We still are attached to these labels or categories as if they had real meaning for the functional design of educational programs. It is true that a brain-injured child may behave differently from a mentally retarded child or that a child with cerebral palsy has some problems that are different from a child whose problems are primarily emotional. But the functional problems of all of these children do overlap, as sometimes do the causes of their handicaps, that it seems to me to be foolish to hold to these categories, especially in educational planning. The educational problems that these children have relate to behavioral processes rather than diagnostic categories. Let us take, for example, a child who is diagnosed to be a mental defective. Mental retardation may be the end product and the condition which sets her apart socially but the culpable process with respect to learning may be faulty stimulus reception, disturbed perceptual integration, or distorted symbol codification. Now any one of these conditions may also be the functional culpable agent in a variety of other diagnostic conditions. When we continue to concentrate on the diagnostic category, we mislead ourselves, we misinform public policy, we Balkinize the political power base, and we encourage educators to classify and treat around socially perceived conditions that have little meaning for educational intervention. We also discourage or at least do not provide support for diagnostic services and treatment, attention being given to the functional processes that Ms. Haeussermann reminds us should be the focus of our attention.

If we are to plan effectively for handicapped children's education, recreation, or vocational training, the first and essential task is to analyze the behavior of these children in such functional detail as to inform the intervention process. The second task involves the transformation of these data into instructional, supportive and experiential encounters that complement need — style-functional conditions.

But the tasks of education do not begin and end with the enlightened application of behavioral science knowledge to professional practice. All human efforts must be approached within the context of the political economy of the phenomenon under study. Increasingly, I am convinced that education cannot be fully understood outside of the political economy of education (knowledge of the ways in which power and resources in support of education are distributed and controlled). Education is also not likely to be significantly changed without the active manipulation of that process.

Certainly education of handicapped persons is no exception. Until we are able to intrude with the concerns of the handicapped on the political economy of education and human development and influence that process, the things we talk about here are not likely to come to fruition. To achieve this we will have to break down the barriers of diagnostic group separation and begin to tackle together the functional problems and needs of this varied but in many ways similar population. To look beyond the trees to see the power of this forest without overlooking species that add to its diversity is our task. To utilize that power in support of the diverse needs is our challenge.

Alternative Forms of Care for the Disabled: Developing Community Services

Robert Morris, MSC, DSW

"Community services for the disabled" is a currently popular phrase which has been adopted by so many different types of interest groups that its specific meaning has become blurred. Hospitals and institutions for the disabled are, of course, community facilities in the sense that they are supported by a community, but the current use of the term is usually restricted to those efforts to replace a primary reliance on large-scale institutions with a variety of services provided in a neighborhood. In this definition the term "community services" still includes hospitals; rehabilitation centers; small institutions, such as nursing homes, halfway houses, and day centers; as well as the delivery of services to the homes of disabled persons. Also, the use of the term "care" can be used to mean something other than, or in addition to, active treatment and rehabilitation. I should like to focus upon a definition of *care* which comprises the attention or the assistance which the disabled need *other than* active medical treatment or rehabilitation. For all practical purposes, this requires attention to those circumstances in the conditions of the disabled that require the attention of another person sometime during the day or night if the disabled individual is to survive or to live in conditions which we consider minimally acceptable. I should further like to concentrate the discussion on care or community service directed to the majority of the severely disabled persons who continue to live in a family or family-type setting so that the disability does not produce an unnecessary disruption in normal living patterns through permanent removal to an institution, be it large or small. Cast in these terms, the subject might better be stated as: "How shall we distribute our human service effort to meet the living requirements of the disabled, and how shall we organize these efforts?".

SCOPE AND HIDDEN CHARACTER OF THE PROBLEM

Our approach to community care has been colored by 100 years of confidence which has pervaded our approach to illness. Most of our efforts, organization, and enthusiasm, as well as investment of funds, have been premised upon the view that the conquest of disease itself is progressive. The enormous achievements in the reduction of infant mortality, in the management of infectious disease, and the deferral of death through technologic and nutritional means, have created a sense of confidence that the more we push the boundaries of investigation the closer we come to preventing disease and conquering the physical hazards of existence. Thus, virtually all of our public policy, our voluntary as well as governmental service programs, and our professional services are based on the conviction that we best use our energies to assist the disabled in overcoming their handicaps, if indeed we are not yet able to prevent all of them, so that the individuals can resume a relatively normal way of life *without further assistance from society*. A new awareness of the ecologic and social environment has led to valuable efforts to modify the physical environment of the disabled so that they are better able to function with their disabilities. At bottom, however, both of these approaches assume that social provision has a definite termination after which the disabled person or his family will continue to function without further external assistance. Those who do not quite fit the optimistic view are considered to be relatively temporary failures in the progress of science.

A look at a different body of evidence may lead to a contrary conclusion. The following views about community services lead to a relatively simple thesis: the greater our successes in overcoming acute threats to existence, the greater is the increase in long-term disability and chronic illness in the population. It has been said that living brings us closer to death. Equally, we can say that rescue from physical trauma will probably bring us closer to disability as well. The more we succeed, the more it becomes necessary for society to attend to long-term living requirements of the disabled which require the efforts of other individuals on a long-term, if not permanent, basis. The evidence for this conclusion is pieced together from a variety of incomplete bits of evidence. Most of the information available on disability is organized either around medical diagnoses which do not readily permit disaggregation into functional subcategories or around social services which, in turn, are developed around diagnostic categories which do not permit ready aggregation of evidence across the entire span of disability.

If we take a generic approach to disability, one which regards the common aspects of disability and which aggregates all forms of *severe* disability regardless of age or of etiology, then it appears that long-term, irreversible disability is a significantly growing phenomenon, growing both in incidence and in prevalence.

A recent report of the Social Security Administration [1] indicates that between 1960 and 1970 there was an increase of 225% in the number of Social Security beneficiaries between the ages of 18 and 64 years who suffer from severe, permanent disabilities which prevented the performance of normal major tasks. In this same period, among the total worker beneficiary population, the proportion of the totally disabled increased from 5.3 to 10.1%, nearly double.

A recent attempt [2] to assess the cost of disability finds that nearly $83 billion of health, medical, and transfer expenditures is alloted to the disabled. This includes episodic and acute treatment of health conditions which are diagnostically identified as chronic illnesses as well as disability-triggered income transfers. These sums are distributed as follows: medical, $46.5 billion; income transfers, $34 billion; direct services, $2.3 billion.

Such evidence is, of course, not conclusive and can be explained by a variety of factors: better case finding, liberalization of benefits, more generous administrative or clinical procedures. However, a closer examination of several more specific items suggests that any optimistic view that scientific advances will reduce the incidence of disability is premature at best and possibly unwarranted.

1) In 1937, the Office of Children reported that there were 24 severely crippled children per 10,000 population who were beneficiaries of that program. In 1957, the same program reported 47 crippled children per 10,000 population with like conditions.

2) In 1960, the Social Security Administration made annual lifetime payments to 100,000 permanently disabled children of Social Security beneficiaries – those permanently disabled before the age of 18 which rendered them incapable of economic employment after that age. In 1972, this number, an accumulative one, had increased to 300,000.

3) There is increasing evidence of a perceptible increase in the number and proportion of infants who are born with severe malformations or with early life-endangering conditions. For example, our success in keeping alive children born with very low birthweight or with severe respiratory distress symptoms has been accompanied by evidence that a significant proportion of such children are likely to survive with permanent central nervous system defects (6% of those with low birthweights and 19% of those with severe respiratory symptoms). While much has been made of the very great success in conquering the disabilities of poliomyelitis, there has been no comparative study which seeks to balance such dramatic gains with the kind of equally dramatic losses which would permit us to assess whether, overall, there is increase or decrease in disability.

4) Finally, since 1900, the improvements in infant mortality, nutrition, and economic well-being have greatly enlarged the proportion of older persons who now survive into their 70th and 80th years. By current projections, while the total

population is expected to grow by only 10% in 10 years, the population over 75 years of age is expected to grow by 22%. It is this over-75 population which contains a very large reservoir of permanent disablement and long-term chronic disability, and which represents the largest consumption of hospital or long-term care resources.

Since 1940, we have found ways to keep young adults, who break their spinal cords in accidents, alive for decades although they are permanently paralyzed from neck or waist down. In 1939, such patients usually died within a year or two [3].

5) In the aggregate, between 6 and 25 million persons not in institutions may be in the scope of our discussion. The committee planning the 1976 White House Conference on Disability estimates 35 million American citizens to be disabled. This is undoubtedly a journalistic exaggeration which includes relatively minor vision and hearing handicaps. But even a more conservative estimate, limited to persons who are unable to perform their major normal functions in life, finds an estimated 6 million persons of all ages not in institutions but who need another person's regular attention over time [4]. This need does not negate the need to normalize their social acceptance as to work, education, love, etc.

The problem of developing community services must be attacked with the recognition that there has probably been a radical shift in the nature of our health problem: a shift accounted for by 1) technical capacity to keep alive fragile infants; 2) to keep the young, severely injured alive for decades (spinal cord injuries); 3) to keep older adults alive for years with severe disability.

IMPLICATIONS FOR COMMUNITY CARE

If the problem of community care is to be tackled not from the point of view of single diagnostic categories but rather from a generic approach to disability, we need to shift our perspective away from the current one which is, in oversimplified fashion, as follows. What happens to the disabled person after completing active treatment and rehabilitation is primarily the family's responsibility; if the family network breaks down, it's the residual or occasional awkward case which requires social intervention.*

If we are to approach the subject of community services from a truly comprehensive and generic point of view, 3 gross categories of social circumstances need to be reckoned with: 1) the disabled person with close family ties and willing family caretakers; 2) the disabled with available families who have difficulty or

---

*Such a generic approach is foreshadowed by the adoption of the term "developmental disability." Although the term today refers primarily to a limited number of diagnostic categories, primarily affecting children, many of the disabilities of old age are equally developmental in their character.

reluctance in providing care; 3) disabled persons without family ties (the increase in the proportion of American women who never marry or who are divorced for long periods of time or who are widowed; the increase in families with only one child or none; as well as the well-publicized mobility of American families all suggest that this category of adult without significant family ties has been increasing and will probably be increased in the future).

The present effective state of service organization is one in which perhaps 95% of our social health investment goes to pay for hospital, nursing home, and medical and treatment services. This is clearly true for Medicare and, although not required by legislation, is practically true for Medicaid where the provisions of public assistance for the poor have generally made it easier for these funds to be used for nursing homes rather than for other forms of care for the disabled. Relatively minor exceptions to this rule are found in Workmen's Compensation and in the Veterans' Administration, each of which pays benefits for both medical and for physical personal care for select populations. This direction of our public fiscal investment has determined effectively the delivery of our social provision for the disabled, which is predominantly for relatively short-term attention following treatment on the premise that individuals or families will assume care responsibilities in a relatively short period of time.

The major exception to this general statement may be our investment in income maintenance programs, in which it is assumed that an individual unable to perform in the labor force is entitled to subsistence income replacement and that he/she will survive adequately with a replacement of less than their normal earnings. These income programs make no provision for the *additional* costs of securing someone's help for personal care, costs which persons who have otherwise adequate basic income would have a hard time meeting. Such additional costs are *not* covered by present medical or home health services and are only partly covered for perhaps 50% of our at-risk population in nursing homes. Old Age and Survivors Disability Insurance and Supplementary Security Income are examples of the limitations of an income replacement program.

Neither of our major policy approaches, therefore, takes into account the growing proportion as well as number of persons who, with their disability, require continuing, long-term, perhaps permanent attention from another individual, the costs of which are in excess of normal living expenditures for the well, able-bodied individual or family.

THE RELATIONSHIP BETWEEN FAMILY AND SOCIAL PROVISION

In this situation, it has been commonplace for our medical and health systems to rely primarily upon family networks for the provision of care beyond the relatively short period of assistance now available through Medicare and Medicaid. Where this breaks down, the reliance is placed upon institutional care in various forms, much of it obscured by the nicer sounding term of "community institution," such as the nursing home or some other congregate living residence smaller in scale than the large chronic hospital.

This state of affairs is obviously a topsy-turvy one, for the primary satisfactory thrust of a public policy or of a community program would be one which builds first on the base of family and normal living arrangements, with *any form* of institutional care, be it large or small, a care arrangement of *last* resort. (Or one reserved for the most severely disabled requiring virtually full-time, continuous attention of another.) Since our arrangements are thus reversed, most of our information about the disabled is unfortunately based upon the condition of those who are now in institutional care, representing perhaps 5% of the total risk population. Very little systematic study has been accumulated over the years about the secular experience of the disabled living outside of institutions.

The crucial role which the family plays and the symbiotic relationship between family and social provision (be it institutional or other) is documented in a recent study completed at Brandeis University [5]. A sample of patients discharged from 4 chronic disease and rehabilitation hospitals, for whom a package of community services was prescribed, was followed for 6 months after discharge. For one of the most crucial areas, assistance with activities of daily living, specific assistance was prescribed in two-thirds of the cases. In 64% of these prescribed cases, families provided the bulk of care and in only 11% did social agencies or health agencies provide any supplemental assistance to families. Chore or household services were prescribed in 81% of the cases, and relatives provided all such assistance in 80% of these prescribed cases.

Of greater significance are the findings concerning the effect of long-term disability on families' willingness and capacity to provide care. Over 70% of the patients discharged to community care had intact family units which had provided care in the past. They had given such care without any external supplemental help at all in most cases. Where this hospitalization was the first, 70% of the families were ready to take the patient and to give all care. Where there had been successive hospitalizations, and no supplemental help to the family, the percentage of willing families dropped by one-half, to 38%.

The thesis must be seriously considered that adequate attention for the severely disabled requires the provision of substantial personal and home-care services, other than psychologic, therapeutic, and rehabilitative, which can supplement and not replace an intact family's willingness to share the burden of long-term care for the severely disabled. An ideal arrangement, tested in some European countries, would provide a large-base foundation of such services supplementing family capacity and parallel to extensive, active, and rehabilitative treatment services. Where family capacity is not present (30% in the Brandeis sample) or erodes beyond rescue, then alternative forms of community services in some type of institutional or group living pattern remain as fall-back arrangements. However, the primary-foundation community services are personal care, chore services, and day-care services to relieve families during the daylight hours.

The exact pattern of relationship between such services and therapeutic facilities and the mechanisms by which a proper mix is achieved between family burden and social provision needs yet to be developed. The burden is much too large to assume that all care of the severely disabled will be provided by some form of public social provision. Similarly, it is equally illusory to assume that all personal care can be provided by families, with public provision concentrated only on active treatment.

RECENT DEVELOPMENTS AND IMPLICATIONS FOR THE FUTURE

This analysis of cure and care mix is now being tested in a number of federally funded experiments. Less well known, perhaps, are some comprehensive community programs which have already begun by local initiative without massive federal support. A number of local programs for the retarded and for the aged have evolved on a demonstration basis wherein one administering agency controls a wide spectrum of home care, day care, chore services, and sometimes extending to protective, small-scale residential accomodations. Such agencies no longer depend on giving one service and then referring cases to others for completing the required cycle of services which a severely disabled person requires. In a recent study of innovations in local social service delivery, 14 concrete services were identified, ranging from testing and counseling through provision of protective services, residential care, and the like [6]. Thirty-one innovative programs were identified, and 18 of the 31 controlled, through direct delivery of purchase, two-thirds or more of these concrete services.

A generic type of program has also begun to emerge. Local public welfare agencies are also beginning to provide a variety of social services without regard to diagnostic category or age (although income limitations are a determining factor). In a recent study of programs in 6 New England states under the new Title XX Amendments to the Social Security Act, it was found that day care, community residential care, homemaker services, or foster care services on such relatively generic bases account for between 50% and 65% of all public social services expenditures in the surveyed states [7].

Such demonstrations of local initiative, however, are based upon the most insecure financial foundations, depending as they do upon annual appropriations in a period of financial stringency. Whether any of these innovations will survive the present constricting financial climate is unclear. Such uncertainty makes it all the more important to seek out more stable ways to finance and to organize such generic caring services.

At least 2 experiments are underway, with federal support, which may represent *the first steps to the future – insuring for the costs of long-term social provision for the disabled*. In Connecticut, Medicare funds are authorized to an experimental agency which has in its own authority the funds and means to pay for any "appropriate" services which a disabled Medicare-eligible person may need, ranging from modest payments to a relative to provide supplementary care at home, through the purchase of extensive homemaker services, all the way to full-time hospitalization. For the first time, a very generous, perhaps too generous, program will test out what happens when a truly comprehensive range of services can be provided for any disabled persons without regard to origin of disability and without regard to fund limitations as between care at home and care in an institution. In Wisconsin, Medicaid funds are being used for similar tests whereby money is available without regard to age, but only for low-income families, for the purchase or direct provision of *any* service which might be considered useful to assist disabled individuals maintain their normal living circumstances.

Such experiments still carry with them some residue of earlier expectation, that somehow individuals will, as a result of these services, be able to provide more of their own care for themselves. But at last a clear test is now underway to identify the consequences of a relatively unconstrained program for funding community care services of any kind, including the reimbursement of services provided by family members.

An insurable basis for community care for the physically disabled contains one risk. Benefit payments to persons may not lead to the requisite mix of care and cure services, since this health "marketplace" may not respond to conventional market incentives. On the other hand, an insurable basis for public policy may hasten the day when we will fund our care programs as securely as we fund our episodic medical treatment programs.

I should like to conclude by suggesting that the true future of community services for the disabled lies in our recognition that long-term disability is here to stay and that it is subject to the same kind of definition that other health services have been subject to for purposes of insurance. In other words, social provision for the long-term disabled can be initially funded through insurance mechanisms in much the same fashion that we now insure for physician and hospital services. We are now nearly at the point where the population at risk and the incidence of risk can be identified and benefit packages relevant to these risks can also be specified.

There is substantial anxiety about the fiscal burden which such an approach would incur. I believe these anxieties are ill founded. We already spend over $100 billion on medical care, 80% of which is allocated in some way to the chronic illness area. Some part of these present expenditures can be better spent in a new mix of cure and care. Perhaps 25% of our present expenditures from health funds (Medicare and Medicaid) for nursing-home care is unwarranted and could be diverted to providing home-delivered services at no increase in cost, and perhaps at some reduction in some cases. In addition, the evidence about inappropriate utilization of inpatient beds and outpatient hospital visits is also extensive. In such cases, there are strong indications that substitution of less costly forms of social provision are acceptable and desirable and would affect medical expenditures in a measurable fashion.

However, this future requires that we accept the inescapable linkage between medical care and social provision for the long-term disabled. Our public policy can no longer invest almost exclusively in medical treatment while ignoring that the success of this treatment produces a subsequent personal, family, and social burden of overpowering magnitude, that of increasing long-term disability. In the end, our public policy must not only rescue lives, but must provide for a minimally decent living in family circumstances for most of those whose lives are thus rescued. We must reassess the distribution of our effort as between treatment and care so that a more equitable balance is restored. To treat and ignore the consequences is indefensible, just as is the attempt to provide care without appropriate treatment. If both cannot be done at the maximum, then some sufficient balance must be struck between them.

We already have demonstrations and experiments which are steps along the road to this path. We also have vast, untapped national experiments in the form of the Veterans' Administration which now provides such care and cure combinations for a limited sector of the population. What is now needed is a comprehensive and systematic attack on disability in its generic form in order to firm up the foundation for an insurance approach to disability which takes into account living as well as treatment and income replacement. To this end, the work to date needs to be furthered by 1) the accumulation of more specific and sharply defined data; 2) the improved design of experiments and their evaluation; and 3) the evolution of policies based upon these data and these experiments in order to frame an appropriate insurance mechanism.

It is not at all clear to me that such work can or should be entrusted to our medical system. Can we ask our hospitals, for example, to *discharge* no disabled patient until he or she is provided the social care I have talked about *and* pays for such care, without passing the "buck" to family or another welfare agency? If we cannot, we clearly need a parallel social support system, with a significant share of present medical dollars being allocated to it.

I doubt if systematic work will proceed rapidly enough unless we have some central clearing mechanism to keep the work proceeding. In the 1920s and the 1930s, the Committee on the Cost of Medical Care, under the able leadership of Michael Davis, provided such a core for the whole evolution of our views about health insurance. Perhaps the time has come when a comparable, scientific committee of interested persons can organize themselves to pursue the subject of disability in modern society.

REFERENCES

1. Lerner, P. R.: Social security disability applicant statistics. Office of Research and Statistics, Social Security Administration (1970).
2. Worral, J.: Preliminary report of a study of the economic cost of disability. Rutgers University. (Mimeograph.)
3. Eggert, G. M.: Post-rehabilitation experiences of a population of spinal cord injured veterans. Brandeis University, unpublished doctoral dissertation.
4. Levinson Policy Institute, Brandeis University: Alternatives to nursing home care. Senate Special Committee on Aging, Government Printing Office (October 1971).
5. Eggert, G. M., Morris, R., Granger, C. V., and Pendleton, S.: Community-based maintenance care for the long-term patient. Brandeis University (January 1975) (Mimeograph.)
6. Morris, R., Hirsch-Lescohier, I., and Withorn, A.: Social service delivery systems: Attempts to alter local patterns 1970–1974. Brandeis University (January 1975). (Mimeograph.)
7. Hirsch-Lescohier, I., Akula, L., and Morris, R.: Review of initial Title XX plans in Region I, HEW. (Research in progress, Brandeis University).

Influence of Litigation on the Lives of the Developmentally Disabled: A Preliminary Report

Kathleen G. Ursin, MS

"The squeaky wheel gets the grease," is a well-known phrase that has too often proved true in social systems faced with the problem of allocating scarce resources. With increasing frequency, it is the vocal and often disruptive elements, unafraid to make their demands known to an unaware and sometimes apathetic bureaucracy, that initiate improvements and secure program funding. In the labor field, for example, it is the striking unions that accomplish cost of living increases, arbitration settlements, and more adequate pension funds. Until prison riots erupted, sometimes inhumane conditions in our prisons went unattended and unheeded. Too often rights are protected only when it is made painfully aware to society that these rights are being violated. This awareness can often best be fostered by the people actually experiencing the deprivation in conditions brought about by the lack of basic human rights.

What happens however to those individuals in our society who cannot achieve these goals on their own behalf? Who can help the powerless, the naive, the sometimes not fully competent segments of our society who are often unaware of the existence of their rights, or who are not sufficiently articulate to explain their needs fully? The judicial system, the system of laws and the opportunities which it provides for redress of grievances, can provide a forum for the articulation, examination, and potential solution to such problems. Can or should courts, however, provide the continuous monitoring service that is often necessary to assure that decisions reached in a court of law are implemented?

In speaking with you today, I would like to examine some of the seminal lawsuits in the area of rights of the handicapped which have great implications for the developmentally disabled. These include the *Wyatt* v. *Stickney* suit in Alabama dealing with right to treatment issues and the *PARC* v. *Commonwealth of Pennsylvania* and *Mills* v. *Board of Education* suit in the District of Columbia which deal with right to education questions. I will discuss briefly the background of these cases and then explore some of the difficulties in the implementation of decisions and make some assessment of the impact that such litigation has had on securing rights for developmentally disabled persons.

The court's role in remedying intolerable treatment and training conditions which can and do exist in public and private, state and local, large and small facilities, must be two-fold in order to be effective. First, it must provide the initial awareness to society at large that the need for change is real and, second, it must act as an implementing force for any standards that it may set. How adequately the judiciary can accomplish these functions, and the problems that arise in trying to do so, have become immediate issues in the right to treatment controversy.

In 1966, in the case of *Rouse* v. *Cameron* [1] Judge Bazelon first spoke for the patient's right to treatment. Mr. Rouse, after being found not guilty on grounds of insanity for carrying a dangerous weapon, was involuntarily confined to a mental hospital. Claiming that he received no medical treatment while he was incarcerated, Mr. Rouse brought a *habeas corpus* action for his release. Judge Bazelon, in granting the order for the court, recognized Mr. Rouse's right to treatment, but based it on a federal statute, the 1964 Hospitalization of the Mentally Ill Act. Judge Bazelon found that the hospital needed to show a "bonafide effort to cure" [2] the patient to justify incarceration.

Five years after the *Rouse* court recognized a right to treatment, a federal district court in Alabama [3] gave this right a Federal constitutional basis. With the establishment of such a constitutional right to treatment, each state may be faced with a challenge to its system of care and treatment for institutionalized individuals. To some extent, the defendants in the *Wyatt* case conceded the constitutional right to treatment issue and, therefore, the court's justification for finding such a constitutionally based right is vague.

In both the *Rouse* and *Wyatt* cases the court found intervention proper and necessary in protecting committed patients, but, after these decisions, some courts are still questioning the threshold issue of whether or not the right to treatment is a justiciable one, in other words, proper subject matter for the courts. For example, in 1972 a Georgia District Court granted no relief in a right to treatment case and found the issue of right to treatment to be nonjusticiable [4]. The justiciability of an issue involves 3 factors: 1) whether judicially discoverable and manageable standards exist by which to measure the rights and duties of the parties; 2) whether judicial resolution of the controversy will comport with due respect for the other departments of government, the legislative and executive branches; and 3) whether courts can effect an adequate remedy. The justiciability question is especially relevant in the right to treatment area because of the involvement with state agencies that is required with any relief granted. By taking the problem out of the domain of the court system, the Georgia District Court placed the burden of relief squarely on the state legislatures. Right to treatment was defined as a political question beyond judicial scope. Ironically, whether the issue is capable of court intervention or not, the legislatures must play a vital role in any permanent relief that is to be accomplished. However, it is the more basic question of the court's right to order the relief that is in question here.

Judicial intervention is always proper where constitutional rights are involved. However, is the imposition of a federal court decree on a state a violation of the principle of comity between state and federal governments? Practically speaking, mandatory relief ordered by the court may best be implemented when intragovernmental bodies are given a chance to choose among alternative remedial measures and select responses which will not interfere with established relationships but which will still be constitutionally sufficient. Nevertheless, if the state fails to act when given this alternative the courts have demonstrated a willingness, as in *Wyatt*, to set standards [5]. This still leaves unanswered, however, the question of whether courts can develop standards which are more adequate and suitable, and by establishing such standards, whether the courts can assure appropriate treatment care.

Right to treatment cases such as *Wyatt* have raised an additional question in terms of the courts' ability to require additional state appropriations for funds for improvements in the mental health system. This question raises the possibility of violations of the 11th Amendment rights of states. Compliance with a court order requiring expenditure of funds are usually directed against state officials and not the state itself, and, therefore, this question is not pertinent. However, it again raises the importance of securing cooperation from the defendants if court-ordered changes are to be realized.

The question of the courts' ability to enforce mandatory injunctive relief is difficult to evaluate. Although recent federal and state cases made clear that difficulties of enforcement will not prevent the issuance of injunctions to protect constitutional rights, the effectiveness and scope of court-ordered remedies must be analyzed.

In the first *Wyatt* decision, for example, the defendants were given 6 months to implement necessary changes which the court had ordered in institutions in Alabama. After 6 months of inaction on the part of mental health officials in the state, the court set about trying to implement its decree by setting both qualitative and quantitative standards for state institutions [6]. Quantitative standards are not only easier to establish but also easier to implement. However, because they require an alteration in existing facilities within institutions, they may require the use of state resources for institutional programs and potentially deny such funds to the development of community programs.

In implementing the qualitative rights required in *Wyatt*, such as rights to privacy and dignity, and the right to the least restrictive therapeutic alternative [7], the court found it necessary to appoint a committee for each state facility to advise and assist patients who allege the infringement of their legal rights [8]. These human rights committees, as they were called, were to serve as the "eyes and ears" of the court during the implementation process. They were responsible for monitoring the changes in the institution and ensuring that the constitutional rights of the residents were being observed. Although in theory these human rights committees provided the "squeaking wheel" for initiating further judicial intervention and relief, their lack of full-time staff to continuously monitor the institutions, the absence of mental health experts among their membership, and the absence of any legal powers greatly diminished the relief they could offer [9].

Right to treatment litigation serves to undermine much existing mental health legislation, as well as the once perceived, if not still perceived, role of the mental health institution in relieving society of the necessity of caring for its impaired persons in the community. Dr. David Mechanic of the University of Wisconsin, in discussing the *Wyatt* decision, has commented that because of this function of mental hospitals it is unlikely that they will ever be abolished completely. Institutions, he feels, serve as a useful mechanism for social control and, therefore, are found to be valuable to the social order. Therefore, he states that the courts and the legislatures ". . . will attempt to adapt to external attack by modifying the more abusive practices, by providing greater opportunity for review, and by attempting to improve those more visible conditions that arouse public concern. . . . Although litigation creates temporary discomfort, it is difficult without constant surveillance to insure that the gains achieved can be maintained in the future." He states further that "no matter how astute the litigants or how passionate the court, the long-term quality of our hospitals, our rehabilitation institutes, our schools and our society generally depends on more fundamental decisions made through the legislative process" [10].

In reviews of the *Wyatt* decision, 3 main faults of the decree have been articulated [11]. Even though the court had instituted fact-finding committees within the suspect institutions, the court's ability to obtain information about whether or not compliance was taking place was greatly impaired by the self-serving aspect of any information received from the defendants, and the sporadic, noncontinuous information gathering functions of the human rights committees.

The decree itself contained possibly conflicting requirements, such as the transition from institutionalization to the least restrictive alternative possible coupled with the restructuring of institutions to make them more humane. While the first requirement calls for a move to deinstitutionalization, the latter asks for an improvement in present conditions. This conflict, as mentioned previously, could result in the use of resources to fulfill the requirement of improving the institution, yet would leave no resources for the process of deinstitutionalization.

The scope of the decree presents a further problem. For example, what would be done if abuses not contemplated in the original complaint are uncovered in the course of implementation? In fact, this situation has arisen, calling for the necessity of further litigation and for the implementation of further costly study and change. Indeed, nearly 5 years later, aspects of the case are still being litigated. Part of the reason for this continued litigation is that the human rights committees had no legal powers to implement necessary changes.

Any court action has inherent time-consuming features that detract from the use of the court as the "solver" of problems. The judicial implementation process is basically defective in providing the type of immediate comprehensive relief required in right to treatment cases. Like a parent who relies on his child's respect for his authority in seeing that orders are obeyed, the court must rely on legislative compliance if its orders are to be implemented. Indeed, there must be some cooperative aspect to each settlement between plaintiffs and defendants if decrees of the courts are to be effectuated [12].

If the courts are ill equipped to deal with implementation problems, then an alternative model should be developed which would address the problem. Hoffman and Dunn have recently proposed such a model consisting of 4 major components: 1) a rule-making board to promulgate regulations and ensure the preservation of statutory and consititutional rights of patients; 2) case-deciding personnel (treatment evaluators), who would conduct informal counsel proceedings following alleged violations of patient's rights; 3) a legal-aid service to inform patients of their rights and act as their attorneys in proceedings before treatment evaluators and other bodies; and 4) a panel of mental health judges specializing in litigation of mental health issues. Jurisdiction would include initial and subsequent commitments, and appeals from the decisions of treatment evaluators [13]. Two states, Pennsylvania and Michigan, have suggested an administrative program, although not as comprehensive as the one detailed above. Neither of these proposals has been passed into law.

The Hoffman-Dunn model presents considerable difficulty in implementation from several standpoints. However, the component which could present the greatest problem is the establishment of the panel of mental health judges. This is not to say that the idea has no merit. Indeed, many abuses of these civil commitment procedures are attributable in part to the failure of the courts to seriously hear the evidence presented to them and a tendency to accept whatever advice is given to them by expert witnesses. If courts are to continue hearing these cases, they must develop an increased ability to make judgments concerning mental illness and mental retardation on the basis of the facts, with greater awareness of the limits of medical and psychologic evidence.

Even the suggested administrative solutions are basically adversarial judicial proceedings to obtain relief. Where one of the parties is incompetent to engage on an equal footing in the two-party system of law, what remedies can we offer to close the gap? In a recent paper Nader and Singer state that "one of the greatest challenges facing the legal profession is to create forums that can resolve disputes between distant, unequal parties with both fairness and credibility" [14]. They suggest that a third-party system of ombudsman or arbitrators be established to create some sort of formal grievance procedure to deal with complaints. Arbitration and mediation have been used successfully in a number of areas to resolve disputes. It has been effective, however, only when groups of individuals, such as employees, ban together to form cohesive groups. With the increasing development of consumer advocate groups, parent groups, and organizations of friends of disabled persons, particularly the developmentally disabled, this model gains more and more credibility as a potential solution to problems. In any area in which disputes now go unresolved or consume scarce judicial resources, arbitration and mediation promise possibilities for solution, particularly when parties deal with one another on a continuing basis. This process could apply to all institutions — that is, not only the hospital setting as dealt with in *Wyatt* but to the school as an institution as dealt with in the seminal litigation in *PARC* v. *Pennsylvania* and *Mills* v. *Board of Education*.

These 2 major cases were decided in 1972. *PARC* v. *Commonwealth of Pennsylvania* and *Mills* v. *Board of Education* made clear that where the state, or in the *Mills* case the District of Columbia, statutorily required public education for children, then the state must provide free public education for all children, including the handicapped.

The *PARC* suit was brought against school officials in Pennsylvania for exclusion of retarded children based on 4 then-existing state statutes. These state statutes were attacked on 2 grounds: 1) that they violated due process by not providing for a notice or a hearing before a retarded child was excluded from education, and 2) that the statutes did not grant the plaintiffs equal protection because the premise upon which they were based, namely that retarded children are uneducable and untrainable, lacks a rational basis in fact.

As in the *Mills* case, the parties agreed that a right of education existed for these children and a consent agreement was entered into in order to formulate relief for the plaintiffs. The Pennsylvania attorney general issued official opinions to make clear that the state statutes in question were not meant and could not be used to deny or expel retarded children from public education. In conclusion, the agreement stated that the defendants would formulate a plan ". . . to commence or recommence a pre-public program of education and training for all mentally retarded persons" [15]. The court issued an injunction against applying the state statutes, other than as provided by the agreement, and appointed masters to oversee compliance with the consent agreement.

The *Mills* case was broader than *PARC* in that it included in its class of plaintiffs all exceptional children. Again, the issues involved were failure to provide publicly supported education and training to exceptional children, and exclusion of exceptional children from regular public school classes without affording them due process of law. As in *PARC,* the defendants conceded the obligation to provide education to handicapped children. A consent agreement was also signed in this case, but initial compliance was extremely slow. A further hearing was held by the court to examine the question of delay in implementation and, at that time, the court refused to accept lack of funds as an appropriate barrier to compliance. The court set up a time period for implementation and squarely placed the burden of compliance on the board of education. Unlike the court in

PARC, the *Mills* court did not appoint masters in the District of Columbia. The defendants themselves were made the prime implementing force. Continued lack of compliance with implementation orders, however, necessitated that Judge Waddie again call the defendants back into court, and subsequently appointed a master in the District of Columbia in 1975.

It is important to remember that even where the defendants, state boards of education, agreed that a fundamental right to education existed and cooperated in formulating a process for implementation, serious problems in implementation have arisen and continue to present themselves.

The *PARC* agreement had 4 basic elements: 1) identification of the class of children to be covered; 2) provision to every retarded child of a free public program of education and training appropriate to his learning capacity; 3) hearings and periodic reevaluation of all retarded children at least every 2 years; and 4) notice to parents before changing the assignment or status of any retarded child in the school [16].

The necessity of finding the children and providing appropriate education led Pennsylvania to devise 2 plans: COMPILE, the Commonwealth Plan for Identification, Location, and Evaluation of Mentally Retarded Children, and COMPET, the Commonwealth Plan to Educate and Train Mentally Retarded Children.

The COMPILE program consisted of a massive advertising campaign to locate the children who had been excluded from education and needed help. Unlike the right to treatment class of plaintiffs, who were all institutionalized or recorded as patients in hospitals, the *PARC* decision forced the State of Pennsylvania to make an all-out effort to find children who had never been recorded or been known to be retarded.

A second aspect of COMPILE required evaluation of the child before placement. The evaluation called for included psychologic testing, review of the child's educational status, and an inquiry into the child's family history [17]. The process was time consuming and involved extensive coordinating. In districts with large numbers of previously excluded children, time, personnel, and resources were too limited to effectively fulfill COMPILE's demands. The necessity of both reevaluating children previously placed in special classes and providing evaluations for students never before in the educational system placed such a burden on the local district that reevaluation often meant little more than mere routine affirmation of prior decisions.

COMPET concerned itself with providing appropriate education for the retarded child. To meet this requirement, a total reevaluation of the education and services provided up to the time of the *PARC* decision and preparation to meet the increase in the number of children who would need to be covered in the future under the *PARC* decision had to be undertaken. The term "appropriate education" does not necessarily mean a continuation of present programs augmented only to meet the increased number of students. COMPET, or any program like it, in order to be effective in providing appropriate education to each child, must be an ongoing innovative process. It is obvious, therefore, that the time, money, and expertise necessary to accomplish this type of a program required by a court decree is the major barrier to its implementation. The new children discovered by the COMPILE program, the children already in daily special education classes and temprorary or noninstitutionalized educational programs, were joined by a third class of children, those in state schools and hospitals who also came under the *PARC* decree. Under the terms of the consent agreement, the educational program was to be provided for these children by the Commonwealth Department of Public Welfare, under the supervision of the Commonwealth Department of Education. Although cooperation between the 2 departments was expected, organizational and financial problems arose, leading to a slow-down in implementation.

This organizational mix-up appeared again in enforcing the right to education in private facilities. These facilities were licensed by the Welfare Department, but implementation of educational services was in the hands of the Department of Education. If educational programs were found inadequate and the school or facility refused to adopt a certain standard set by the Department of Education, the only remaining alternative was to close the facility and have the children sent to public schools. Where the public schools were overcrowded and not as well equipped as the private facility might be, parents actually fought the forced change. Although their actions may not have contributed to effectuating long-term solutions, the despair of the parents for the education of their children was understandable.

To say that cooperation existed between the defendants and the plaintiffs in both the *Mills* and *PARC* cases does not mean to suggest that resistance did not exist. Many local school boards, faced with the primary burden of implementation, resisted in the name of politically popular economy drives. Court orders in education suits have not addressed money questions and have left the responsibility for securing the funds necessary to implement the decree to those officials charged with providing education in the state. This has resulted in the cases having a profound impact on normal and special education program administrators, school authorities, and state authorities who must reallocate or redistribute resources from which their program authorizations are drawn.

One prime example of increased levels of funding required under a decree such as *PARC* is that the cost of each due process hearing has been estimated by Pennsylvania officials to be $500. This is equal to one-half the amount spent on the education of the average Pennsylvania child each year [18].

Four monitoring mechanisms were set up by the Pennsylvania court in the *PARC* decree. The first of these was the appointment of masters. Two masters were appointed by the court to approve state proposals for the identification, evaluation, and placement of the children. These same 2 masters were also responsible for hearing complaints, pressing for judicial action against noncomplying officials, and ordering the appropriate persons to testify at hearings. Although these masters provided a central and neutral monitoring device for the court, they did not prove to be completely effective. Both masters were able to devote only part of their time to such duties. As is the problem with many court directives, the court realized that the major burden of implementation must be accepted and carried out by the defendants. The court's reluctance to interfere with state agencies until it became blatantly necessary resulted in many delays in the implementation process. The final weapon of the court, to confront the state legislature by demanding appropriation of funds or institution of legislation, would only have created more problems and delays in implementation.

A second monitoring device set up by the court in the *PARC* decree was the establishment by the Pennsylvania Department of Education of the Right to Education Office. This office was given the responsibility of overseeing the implementation of the consent agreement. However, the office encountered funding problems and, because it was only a temporary agency, it could not provide the continuous monitoring necessary for the ongoing implementation process. Because the office was not independent but linked to the Bureau of Special Education, it developed political problems as well. For example, all statements or policies issued by the Right to Education Office were subject to approval by its parent organization.

A third monitoring device set up by the court was the establishment of local task forces in each educational district. Although these groups were in the districts and closer to the day-to-day implementation process, they lacked effectiveness because their role was advisory only. Furthermore, members of these task forces were selected not by local representation, but by directors of the intermediate school districts.

The fourth monitoring device utilized was the establishment of hearings to ensure procedural due-process rights of children. Formal hearing requirements assured parents the right to a hearing upon initial school placement, after any program change, and after 2 years of special class assignment. Prior to the hearing, parents were given the opportunity to examine school records on which recommendations were based and to retain counsel if necessary. Parents, furthermore, had a right to an open or closed hearing, and were given the opportunity to question all school personnel involved in the decision.

Although in theory this is sound procedural due process, in practice, because of a lack of trained hearing officers and no system by which to inform hearing officers of each other's decisions, this system was far from ideal. Contradictory decisions led to the inability to foresee the outcome of the case, and lack of written and distributed precedents did not help parents in their preparation for hearings. Since the *PARC* decision, the formal hearing system has been slightly modified. Solely technical disputes are now resolved by less formal, prehearing sessions. Additionally, an appeal process which leads to court review of hearing decisions has been devised. Although the hearing process does have some disadvantages, primarily the contrary result brought about by lack of communication and exchange of transcripts between hearing officials, the system is an improvement over the total lack of due process previously accorded the special child. Some merits of the system, in addition to the provision for due process, are that the threat of a hearing and the high cost of conducting such a procedure previously mentioned may be useful political tools for both schools and parents. Thus, without a hearing ever taking place, an individual case could be resolved.

The *Mills* implementation plan included the 3 essential elements of *PARC*, ie identification, evaluation of placement, and due process requirements. The major difference between these 2 decisions, however, was that *Mills* encompassed all exceptional children and did not provide the strict implementation guidelines given in *PARC*. Instead, 9 levels of educational programming were specified in the *Mills* decision: levels 1–3 provided for regular classrooms with special supportive help for the handicapped child; level 4 served the home-bound or hospitalized child by providing visiting instructors; level 5 placed the moderate problem child in "noncategorically compensatory learning centers" away from home on a half-time basis; level 6 created classes for visually impaired and trainable retarded youngsters which were to be conducted in regular schools; level 7 addressed the blind, deaf, severely retarded, physically handicapped, or emotionally disturbed children who were placed temporarily or permanently in special schools; level 8 included the children who would profit from therapeutic day-care programs at mental health clinics; and level 9 provided for those children for whom no appropriate public school placement was possible to receive tuition grants to private schools [19].

This programming function was essentially covered by the COMPET program in the *PARC* case and not detailed in the consent agreement. By detailing the educational programs in the court decree, some of the flexibility inherent in the COMPET plan was forfeited, but implementation should have been smoother. However, this was not the case. Since the court did not initially appoint masters in the *Mills* case, provisions for reporting to the court and keeping data were lacking. The absence of the masters' monitoring function in *Mills* hampered implementation severely. Furthermore, the coordination between departments working toward implementation was poor, and those departments required to engage in joint action maintained little contact.

Finally, the due-process hearings ordered by the court, although similar to those ordered in *PARC*, were always closed to the public and had little procedural formality, giving them the appearance of arbitration seminars rather than legal proceedings. This would not necessarily have been unfavorable had the arbitration been going on between equal parties.

Although both the *PARC* and *Mills* decisions have presented problems and demonstrated the limitations in a court's power, they open up a new frontier for the handicapped — the right to education. They have caused the emergence of new state legislation, frequently enacted in response to litigation but often enacted because of an increasing awareness of problems in this area. Although such legislation is not wholly a result of beneficence or altruism on the part of legislators, it has resulted in greater educational opportunities for developmentally disabled children.

Thomas Gilhool, the plaintiff's attorney in the *PARC* case, lists 4 potential uses for litigation:

> First, citizens may use litigation in order to secure certain substantive rights, in this case access to free public education for all. Second, litigation may be used to create a new place, a new forum, where citizens may turn to enforce their rights and perhaps create new rights. . . . Third, the courts may be used to bring to the attention of the public — the public at large, legislators, decision makers, the ordinary citizen — certain facts that have not had great visibility before. In the right to education cases, for example, the essential fact that all children are capable of benefiting from an education would be brought out. Fourth, the courts may be used by a citizen, as indeed may any other means of petitioning the government for redress of grievances, to express himself, to act out, to tell others who and what he is or in another sense, to redefine, change, or alter his notion of himself [20].

While Gilhool spoke to the possibilities of litigation, the courts, as described previously, are still handicapped in many respects. In the cases outlined, it is apparent that courts are constantly hampered by their difficulties in shaping disputes, controlling resources, selecting among policy alternatives, and monitoring and revising rulings. The necessity of using more than one governmental agency to implement court decisions creates the problems of coordinating activities and unraveling agency bureaucracies, problems that cannot be solved by the courts themselves. Often court decrees can provide temporary change, but are insufficient in themselves to bring about more than a narrow, short term result [21].

Permanent system-wide change is not secured, however, by simply passing a law or writing regulations. In a recent article [22], Thomas Ehrlich, president of the Legal Services Corporations, has made the case for guarding against "legal pollution" — the "thickening layer of legalism which surrounds our lives." He contends that ". . . the basic cause of legal pollution is . . . too much law. Much of the problem is rooted in the public expectations that adjudication is the answer to every dispute and that a statute or regulation is the solution to every unmet need." He offers a number of potential solutions to the problem of legal pollution which include some of those suggested by Hoffman and Dunn [13] and Nader and Singer [14]. They include: 1) removing from the judicial area matters that can be solved by other means; 2) developing procedures to fit the problem as an adversary situation is not always essential; 3) developing "legal impact statements" to accompany legislation; and 4) law training for the public designed to ". . . reduce the aura of mysticism that surrounds the law."

Ehrlich concludes with the following observation:

Faced with so much legal pollution, the temptation of many is to favor disenfranchising from the legal system those without muscle to push... The temptation must be resisted if we really believe, with Learned Hand, that "to keep our democracy, there must be one commandment: Thou shalt not ration justice."

ACKNOWLEDGMENTS

I wish to acknowledge the assistance of Jeannette Cardia, University of Notre Dame/Notre Dame Law School, 1976 and James Albert, University of Notre Dame/Notre Dame Law School, 1975 in the preparation of this paper.

REFERENCES

1. 373 F. 2d 451 (1966).
2. 373 F. 2d at 456.
3. Wyatt v. Stickney, 325 F. Suppl. 781 (M.D. Ala. 1971).
4. Burnham v. Department of Public Health of the State of Georgia, 349 F. Suppl. 1335 (N.D. Ga. 1972).
5. 325 F. Supp. 781 (M.D. Ala. 1971).
6. Wyatt v. Stickney and the right of civilly committed mental patients to adequate treatment. Harvard Law Review 86:1297–1306, 1973.
7. The Wyatt case: Implementation of a judicial decree ordering institutional change. Yale Law Review 84:1342–1343, 1975.
8. Wyatt v. Stickney, 344 F. Suppl. 373 (M.D. Ala. 1971).
9. 344 F. Suppl. 373 (M.D. Ala. 1971).
10. 344 F. Suppl. 373 (M.D. Ala. 1971).
11. Yale Law Review, 84, p. 1362.
12. Mechanic, D.: The right to treatment: Judicial action and social change. Unpublished monograph prepared for conference on Rights of the Mentally Disabled, Wausaw, Wisconsin, September 25–26, 1973, pp. 32–33.
13. Hoffman, P. B., and Dunn, R. C.: Law model for expanding and implementing the mental patient's right to treatment. Virginia Law Review 61:312–313, 1975.
14. Nader, L., and Singer, L. R.: Law in the future: What are the choices? Unpublished papers prepared for a conference sponsored by the State Bar of California, San Diego, California, September 12–14, 1975, p. 39.
15. P.A.R.C. v. Commonwealth of Pennsylvania, 343 F. Supp. 279, 288, (E.D. Pa. 1972).
16. Lippman, L., and Goldberg, I. I.: "Right to Education." New York: Teachers College Press, 1973.
17. Kirp, D., Buss, W., and Kuriloff, P.: Legal reform of special education: Empirical studies and procedural proposals. California Law Review 62:64, 1974.
18. Turnbull, H. R., III: Legal aspects of educating the developmentally disabled. National Organization on Legal Problems of Education, Topeka, Kansas, 1975, p. 33.
19. Public Schools of the District of Columbia: Comprehensive plan for special education: An abstract. pp. 3–8, 1972.
20. Gilhool, T. K.: Education: An inalienable right. Exceptional Children 39:597, 1973.
21. Kirp, D., Buss, W., and Kuriloff, P.: Legal reform of special education: Empirical studies and procedural proposals, op. cit., pp. 112–115.
22. Ehrlich, T.: Legal pollution. New York Times Magazine, February 8, 1976, pp. 17, 19, 21, and 24.

The Making of Public Policy: What Others Do With What We Say We Know

Elizabeth M. Boggs, PhD

I am gratified to join in a symposium honoring Paul Lemkau. Dr. Lemkau came onto my horizon in 1954, when I was pursuing the primary sources of the then widely quoted figure of 1% as the prevalence of mental retardation. The National Association for Retarded Children (as it was then called) was preparing background material for its first public information effort, and 2 of us volunteers, under the guidance of Dr. Salvatore DiMichael, were attempting to get at the hard facts. This led us to the Baltimore survey done in 1936 [1] and to the Williamson County, Tennessee study [2]; these were the only 2 detailed mental health studies then available on populations in the United States.

In 1956, 20 years ago and 20 years after the Baltimore survey, Dr. Lemkau, then Director of New York City's Community Mental Health Service, gave the field of mental retardation another boost by preparing an excellent brief summary, in historic perspective, of the state of the art at that time. The paper "Epidemiological Aspects" was presented at a 4-day symposium on *The Evaluation and Treatment of the Mentally Retarded Child in Clinics* [3]. Unfortunately, the proceedings were published in soft cover without a Library of Congress number, and have, therefore, been lost to the cited literature. Aside from the fact that it predated by 2 years the breakthrough in cytogenetics, the conclusions are valid today.* In the mid-1960s Lemkau, at Johns Hopkins, was guiding Imré in his studies of the prevalence of mental retardation in "Rose County," Maryland. In this survey the justice was done which had in part been denied the retarded in 1936 [7, 8].

*Excellent overviews of recent data are provided by Stein and Susser [4, 5] and by Lapouse and Weitzner [6].

It is not irrelevant to the theme of this paper that both the early Baltimore and Tennessee surveys were focused primarily on mental illness; mental retardation and epilepsy each came in as subordinate mental disorders. In both surveys the various diagnoses, such as schizophrenia, alcoholism, psychoneurosis, epilepsy, and so on, were given a rank order. Mental deficiency was almost at the bottom of the list in both reports. When a case was entered in which more than one disorder was present, the primary diagnosis was assumed to be the one highest on the predetermined list. Thus, tabulated entries of 6.8 and 8.2 per 1,000 (respectively) represented only the cases of mental deficiency which were found to be uncomplicated by any other mental disorder. The summary data found in the initial paper [1] were the most often cited results.

Only a careful reading of the original and subsequent papers [9, 10] revealed that when multiple diagnoses were analyzed, these studies showed overall prevalence rates nearly twice the above. Moreover, these rates were based on survey methods which identified only those cases currently known to service agencies. Based on known cases, age-specific rates varied widely, more than was explainable by differential mortality. Later research has shown that the "disappearance" of retarded adults after they leave school is not by any means entirely explained by a less stringent societal definition of mental retardation among adults as compared to youths in school. Many children identified by schools could later be traced to places in the community where they remained handicapped and dependent yet unserved by any agency and hence uncounted as adults (see eg Saenger [11]). Yet in 1950, it was assumed (incorrectly) that nearly all severely and profoundly retarded persons had been admitted to institutions by age 20.

Prior to 1950 both epilepsy and mental deficiency tended to be perceived as subordinate components of the mental illness continuum, stigmatized even in that context by perceptions of incurability and the need for "custodial care." Autism was not yet familiar as a syndrome; cerebral palsy was discussed in the literature, but crippled children's services were long on surgery, hospitals, and "convalescent care" (cf Benison, this volume). After maximum therapeutic benefit was deemed to have been achieved, the child in need of long-term care was likely to be eased over to the mental retardation institutions, as was the mentally ill child who did not make it in the child guidance clinic. Post polio children were the most common group in public school programs for the orthopedically handicapped as late as 1960 [12]. The idea of subclinical brain damage as a cause of retarded academic performance in the absence of gross neuromotor involvement was just beginning to catch on. Mongolism and cretinism were spoken of in one breath, and neither was very common in adult populations, even in institutions.

I make this recitation partly to point out that there have been some changes in the actual prevalence of some of the component conditions among disabilities originating early in life, but more importantly to stress that our perceptions of them have changed. Our perceptions have implications for public policy.

Public policy is made by many kinds of people. Its raw materials are values, soft facts, hard facts, and contingencies, including political contingencies. Soft facts include perceptions based on hunches, oversimplifications, and extrapolations from inadequate data when adequate data are not available. Prospectively most ecologic and social predictions are based on soft facts; indeed, we can confidently predict that some of the most important future efforts of our present actions are not now being predicted at all.

Public policy is being made all the time. Inaction or postponement of a decision is in itself a decision with consequences, foreseeable and unforeseeable, traceable and untraceable. There are critical periods in the trajectory of public policies as in space flights, but the course is less certain.

Public policy is strongly influenced by little known officials in nonelective positions. Most of them are intelligent but busy individuals who have broad responsibilities. Their information (hard facts and soft facts) come to them through successive filters. In the federal government, for example, both in Congress and in the executive branches, there are identifiable communications networks, but there are several interfaces at which considerable loss of signal as well as distortion can take place.

In a recent NBC special report on US foreign policy around the world, a newsman asked Henry Kissinger, "Does *anyone* know how foreign policy is made?" to which Kissinger smilingly replied, "*I* know how foreign policy is made." And so he may, but it is doubtful that many other incumbent Cabinet officers really know how policy decisions are made in their respective departments.

HEW, for instance, has a fairly clear line and staff table of organization. ("Line" tends to be civil service and "staff" is often short term, less than 2 years.) The interface is defective. The "program managers" are frequently not consulted as to the consequences which they can foresee to a certain policy decision made at the secretarial or assistant secretarial level. Staff are chosen for generic skills rather than for in depth grasp of special issues. They frequently move on before they find out where lie all the things they wanted to know but were afraid to ask.

Like other departments, HEW does have vast repositories of relatively hard facts, as well as the capacity to add to that pool. It spends maybe a $1 billion a year on evaluation and policy analysis, yet loss of specificity along the way to utilization (if any) is inevitable. For example, in HEW, many studies are contracted out often to private research institutes, which live on these contracts, rather than to universities, which are currently seen as having too high an overhead. Each contractor is expected to provide an executive summary of his findings. This is then further abstracted in-house, with special attention to those portions which appear to bear on currently identified issues. Expressions of public opinion and estimates of political fallout are also taken into account. At the same time issues are being consolidated, and data are being aggregated and summarized.

Decision papers are prepared, which are indeed "briefs." On the bottom line are several proposed options for executive selection. It is hard to set up a multiple-choice set of such options, each briefly described, which will adequately exhaust a complex issue, and a secretary may be left unaware of options not presented to him.

Even these processes may be aborted when microdecisions which seem important to us here are swept into macrodecisions somewhere between the secretary, the Office of Management and Budget (OMB), and the domestic policy staff at the White House. Part of Ford's macropolicy (like Nixon's) is to return more of the decision making in public human services delivery to the states. Knowing that general revenue sharing will probably be continued but not much expanded by Congress, the administration recently proposed consolidation of a large array of categorical programs into 4 block grants to states. Block grants are also sometimes referred to as special revenue sharing. The consolidations are proposed under the headings of 1) health, 2) education, 3) social services, and 4) food and nutrition.

In the health field a broad decision was made to fold in direct project grants, along with Medicaid, and a variety of formula grants for health and mental health planning and services, all totaling about $10 billion at current rates of spending. It was also decided not to fold in the well-identified cluster of health professions education programs — capitation to medical schools, nurse training, allied health professionals, etc most of which flows to universities. However, that portion of the maternal and child health program — currently on the order of $20 million — which goes toward training of health professionals to serve handicapped children was proposed for consolidation. These funds presently support interdisciplinary training in a limited number of centers of excellence such as the Kennedy Institute at Johns Hopkins or the Developmental Evaluation Clinic at Children's Hospital in Boston. According to Assistant Secretary of Health, Theodore Cooper, under the President's proposal, it would be up to the 50 states and the District of Columbia to decide whether, and if so how, to continue support to the 21 such existing university centers in 17 states, given the fact that the states would be permitted to spend only 5% of their total grant on all supportive activities, such as comprehensive health planning, data gathering, construction, and personnel development (including training) of all kinds. A similar submergence was proposed for demonstrations and training in special education into the educational services block grant.

To add insult to our injury, all components of the Developmental Disabilities (DD) program, formula grant, project grants, and university training grants, were also proposed for consolidation into the health grant. This move was strongly opposed by the Assistant Secretary for Human Development, in whose office the developmental disabilities programs are now administered. Only a small fraction of DD funds finance health services, and in Congressional budgeting, DD is classed with nonhealth expenditures.

I hasten to add that Congress is not buying the health block grant idea, even though governors favor it, but the process by which this proposal was put together casts some light on the making of public policy [13].

Congress also processes information in the course of decision making. Its approaches tend to be microscopic rather than macroscopic, partly because the committee system has been, and indeed still is, a very decentralized bureaucracy. The establishment of the Congressional Budget Office (CBO) and the enactment of the Budget and Impoundment Control Act represent the first major effort to deal with macropolicy in the economic and social sphere. The full effect has not yet been felt. A second less dramatic but significant development was the establishment of the Office of Technology Assessment (OTA) and the expanding role of the General Accounting Office (GAO), which now conducts program audits as well as fiscal reviews. Until recently technology assessment (TA) has been primarily directed to ecologic concerns, such as the impact of the Alaskan pipeline or insecticides, but recently the National Science Foundation funded a TA study at Texas Tech University to look into the way in which new engineering and social technologies will be likely to change the milieu of the disabled.

The establishment of CBO, OTA, and GAO reflect Congressional interest in commanding its own information sources, independent of both the administration and the most obvious lobbies. Indeed, since the mid-1960s, Congress has moved far in carving out an independent role in policy formulation. At this time its values relative to the handicapped are in large measure consonant with those most commonly espoused by many consumers and some providers. It endorses equal opportunity for the handicapped, including the severely handicapped, and perceives that this entails extra resources. It lacks specific information on optimal use of such resources. As Edmund Gordon (this volume) has pointed out vis-a-vis education, Congress still believes in science most of the time, but does not always recognize its uses [14]. Congressmen need to understand, for example, why a project on teaching mothers to play with their children is not a colossal waste of money.

It is only realistic to recognize that the principal assimilators of this kind of information are not the elected members but their numerous "staffers." It was recently estimated that Congress employs some 17,000 people as staff, or about 30 staffers per member. Some of these are personal staff and some are committee staff, responsive in greater or lesser degree to the particular interests of the committee chairman and members. Although anonymity is their cult, it also is possible to trace significant decisions affecting our interests to the personal interventions of individual staff members whose sensitivity was heightened by personal experience, direct or vicarious. Moreover, although lawyers tend to predominate, some of the country's most able young political, social, and health scientists serve in these anonymous roles.

Congress has certainly responded to the more tangible results of recent research related to the prevention of handicapping conditions in children; we have programs for the prevention of rubella, measles, lead poisoning, and the like. It has also responded to the idea that the lives of young disadvantaged children should be enriched. The result is Head Start and a great enthusiasm (swelled by women's lib) for various day-care programs. The Senate Subcommittee on the Handicapped supports the method of individual tracking of client progress for handicapped individuals, in schools, institutions, and other settings. It is not clear that they understand either the limitations or the costs of representing developmental goals through specific behavioral objectives selected because they are measurable. Congress has, however, mandated the development of a model for a nation-wide evaluation system applicable to developmentally disabled children and adults, based on implementation of an individual program plan for each (P.L. 94-103). A similar provision applies to clients of vocational rehabilitation programs (P.L. 93-516).

Both Congress and the administration are keen on evaluation. Serious workers in this field recognize that expectations often are overly optimistic and that limitations of this technology have not been adequately conveyed to Congress. This is part of what Gurel [15, p. 14] has called "the stereotype of scientific omnipotence."

If science is a needed part of politics, so politics is an inevitable part of science, particularly science applied to human services. In a timely paper, entitled "Evaluation Research in the Political Context," Carol Weiss [16] has said some things that apply equally well to the utilization of professionally legitimated knowledge of other sorts:

> Social scientists tend to see evaluation research, like all research, as objective, unbiased, non-political, a corrective for the special pleading and selfish interests of program operators and policy makers alike. Evaluation produces hard evidence of actual outcomes, but it incorporates as well a series of assumptions; and many researchers are unaware of the political nature of the assumptions they make and the role they play (p. 19).

Some of the highly political assumptions commonly made include the following: 1) Free public education is a right which should be assured through the public schools; it is the child's duty to be educated. 2) Health is a right, but there is no mandate that the individual stay healthy. Health services should be made available through the market place rather than through a public utility, with some cost equalization mechanism added. 3) Social services which are tax supported should be available free to the poor, who should also have priority in access to such services over middle- and upper-class people. Middle-income people should pay for social services in accordance with their ability; currently there is a widespread assumption that state governments should contract with private (including nonprofit) providers for "hard" social services, rather than operate such services directly.

One of the issues which these assumptions raise for us who plan for the developmentally disabled is how to differentiate health services from social services, or education, or rehabilitation, or from bread and butter. There is much board and lodging included in the current health care dollar as Robert Morris (this volume) has pointed out. We are not going to settle that problem in a day, or in 1,000 days, but I would like to suggest that there are some related questions which, if squarely addressed, could somewhat mitigate the dilemma.

I began this paper with a review of some early epidemiologic studies and an intimation of how they reflected the perceptions then held of some of the people we now subsume under the rubric of developmental disability. Epidemiology is concerned with the control of diseases or disorders and relies on the analysis of cumulated data as a heuristic device to lead toward the identification of cause-effect relationships. For this method to be effective, the classification of the disorders must reflect the best guess as to what taxonomy of disease will best map onto a chart of causes. Diagnostic categories have in the past been presumed to offer such a best-guess taxonomy. Regardless of whether this is a reasonably valid assumption with respect to those diagnoses most frequently associated with developmental disabilities, it is quite clear that, from a service point of view, the long-term management of chronic disabilities originating in early life can be better addressed by regrouping on other criteria. Long-term care requires different strategies than primary prevention. Classification which is best for one purpose is not necessarily best for all purposes. This principle is well recognized in law.

The Project on Classification of Exceptional Children conducted under the direction of Nicholas Hobbs [17] addressed the need to approach classification from an ecologic point of view, ie to consider the child's intrinsic deficits in the context of his interaction with his social and physical environment. This theme appears frequently throughout this conference. The Developmental Disabilities Services and Facilities Construction Act of 1970 (P.L. 91-517) was consistent with this consensus in that it focused attention on a group of persons (without regard to age) who *have* severe disabilities which have originated early in life and for which reversal or major remediation appears unlikely.

Some policy makers discuss handicapped children and disabled adults as if they were 2 separate universes. Not all handicapped children become disabled adults, but neither are all disabled adults past the prime of life [18]. In fact if one plots numbers of disabled adults against age at onset of disability, one finds a bimodal curve, with 2 peaks, one in the preschool period and one after 45 [19, 20]. Both phenomena are accompanied by higher mortality. The same factors that cause death also cause disability, but the specific causes at the 2 extremes of age are quite different. Added to the many prenatal chemical, viral, genetic, and physical causes, insults to the immature nervous system in the first few years of life account for the large proportion of permanent handicaps which are in one way or another evidence of cerebral dysfunction. Dr. Strax (this volume) has discussed the perils of adolescence for those so impaired whose cognitive skills and motivation can be developed and who thereby eventually achieve essential social and economic independence. But there are at least half a million adults under 65 who started life as severely handicapped children and who are not able to achieve such self-sufficiency, even in a barrier-free world full of "affirmative action." They are seldom seen in public and are largely ignored when people generalize about the handicapped and their rights. When the economic test is applied to them in adult life, and the population thus defined is examined, most are found to be multiply handicapped with cognitive impairment as a primary or secondary factor.

Most public programs for the handicapped have started with the easy problems; it is more satisfying, professionally and politically, to work with those who are most rapidly responsive to one's ministrations. With them resources can be spread widely, producing many stories of apparent success. Hopefully, one then works down to those with greater needs. The Developmental Disabilities Act, by contrast, is a "bottom-up" model. It was designed to include children and adults with low visibility, as well as others with substantial lifelong disabilities. In it there are no lower limits of eligibility. Its target population is characterized by need for multiple services, beginning early in life, changing with growth but extending in some form into an indefinite future [21, pp. 187-188].

Experience has shown that a person with the combination of functional characteristics specified in the DD Act is at great ecologic risk. Solnit (this volume) has elaborated on this point. The onset of disability (a restriction of life function) early in the developmental period usually entails a variety of secondary effects which are not present when the same impairment is imposed on a mature person. Moreover, differentiation of pathognomonic signs may significantly postdate the initiating event, while in the interim the young child exhibits nonspecific developmental delay. Educational intervention in this period, based on developmental rather than disease-specific criteria, can be critical [22]. Eventual identification of the disability as one likely to persist may trigger a rearrangement of familial and societal priorities for that individual as compared to others, based on unstated principles of triage. Sensing this, the developing personality is at further risk. The needs of the individual will require an extended investment in which the cost-benefit ratio is adverse, unless one places heavy emphasis on psychic benefits [23]; for this and other reasons the individual is likely to be devalued in the perception of both the public and most professionals. It requires an atypical professional orientation for one to be willing to offer supportive social and therapeutic service on an open-ended basis. The program needs in these cases are comprehensive — drawing on health, education, social services, and a variety of subsystems — and cut across disciplinary and other organizational lines. Knowledge of the needed services is not part of the common wisdom, and the affected person and his family may, by the very nature of the disability, lack the know-how to secure such services in the appropriate combination and sequence.

Multiplicity of diagnoses and impairments is likely. The Kuai Pregnancy Study [24] included an analysis of the needs of handicapped children at 2 years of age not merely by diagnosis but by type of special care anticipated. There were 4 groups: 1) minor handicaps requiring little or no special care; 2) handicaps amenable to relatively short-term care; 3) handicaps requiring long-term specialized care and rehabilitation (but not implying social/economic dependency in the adult); and 4) handicaps requiring long-term medical, educational, and custodial care. Of the 23 children (1.3% of the total sample) in group 4, 10 had combinations of physical and mental handicaps, 4 had severe physical handicaps only, and 9 were retarded without significant physical anomaly. Many of the diagnoses in this group were also found in less severe form or in less disabling combinations in the other 3 groups. Group 3 was composed of children with major physical problems, such as heart defects. This distinction matches Anderson's observation (this volume) that children with physical problems which do not affect cerebral function are less globally disabled.

The Kuai study showed that the information obtained by careful individual clinical examinations at the age of 2 was predictive in a collective sense to age 10, especially for the last 2 groups [25]. Some individual children move in and some out of the group to which first assigned but the long-term care cohort does not go away. This finding appears compatible with the British Columbia Register (Miller, this volume).

Even at this early age ICD classification, while important clinically, does not adequately serve a social planning purpose. The further one is removed from the period of onset, the more relevant are the functional aspects of disability as compared to etiology. A look at adults confirms our concern.

Nearly 2 million adults receive Supplemental Security Income because of a disability — defined as "inability to engage in substantial gainful activity" because of a physical or mental condition. We do not yet have detailed current information about the demography or epidemiology of this group since it was redefined by Federal law in 1974, but review of studies made in 1970 under the old aid to the disabled program, administered by the states, tells us some things we should ponder [19]. Although public policy makers frequently subsume the service needs of the adult disabled under those of the elderly, analysis of the 1970 survey data indicates that at least one-third of the current recipients had been disabled since early childhood, many with conditions originating at birth, and that significant impairment of learning ability (whether or not diagnosed as "mental deficiency") is a major impairment even among adults. A comparison of the classification of these adults by *impairment*, with their classification by disease category (ICD) shows that the latter tells us less of what we most need to know when planning for comprehensive but "least restrictive" long-term care [26].

Even these studies do not tell us enough about the extent and nature of social dependence (as reflected, for example, in inability to live alone) or social incompetence (inability to manage one's life with reasonable reference to one's own self-interest), or interpersonal effectiveness, as highlighted by Richardson (this volume). These factors are inadequately documented, with the result that many policy makers fail to take account of the social components in long-term care. This issue has recently been highlighted by Morris (this volume). Especially for those disabled early in life, the *initial* diagnostic label tends to be dominant in determining the sequence of services he will receive, at least until an advanced age. This tendency needs professional reevaluation.

There are some professionals, as well as some political analysts, who will blame the voluntary associations which have grown up in the past 20 years for preserving categorical distinctions. To the extent that this has happened among the disabilities we call developmental, it appears to me to be, at least in part, the result of what we might call *parental imprinting*. The parents are given a diagnosis at birth (or when the child is, say, 2 years old or even 6) along with an indication of how limited are the resources available to help them. If the parents are themselves socially competent, they will conclude that some social action is called for; in 20th century America this means joining with others. What others? To the parents, the most likely colleagues appear as those whose children have been identified as similar, ie having the same *diagnosis*, be it Down syndrome, Tay-Sachs, cystic fibrosis, tuberous sclerosis, or autism. Having once been imprinted, the parents continue to follow and to become identified with the group which they first joined. This group identity, with its potential to combat the individual parent's sense of impotence in the social system, has a particular importance for parents of children with long-term disabilities originating in childhood, because the parent associations, unlike the service system, are organized longitudinally — ie they do not abandon either the disabled person or his family at any age-related point of transition. They are also client oriented, as distinct from discipline oriented, or system oriented. They do not reject the patient when "maximum therapeutic benefit" is achieved, or "potential for employment" is ruled out, or when Blue Cross will no longer cover. The organizations do address comprehensive needs from an individual perspective as these change with age, but they do not restructure their membership along functional as compared to categorical lines. Thus the original imprinting persists. To the extent that public policy is influenced by citizens organized in this way, initial clinical identification has an influence much more far reaching than as a determinant of an immediate treatment regimen.

On the other hand, a completely noncategorical approach to disability can also have detrimental consequences. Submergence of all diagnoses under a single label of handicapped or exceptional can obscure a wide range of differing social and educational (not to mention medical) needs. The most capable among the disabled, especially those first disabled as adults, in asserting their own interests tend to blot out the needs of those less able to speak for themselves. This consumer behavior reinforces the existing professional predisposition to "cream," to give lowest priority to those whose disabilities are the most complex, severe, and of longest duration. Broad categories also tend to be devised to serve the purposes of a single service system, eg education, or welfare, or health, yet management of persons with developmental disabilities must cut across all major delivery systems in an on-going way. In the voluntary association field also, too diffuse a mission leads to perceived ineffectiveness or inequity, which expresses itself in splintering.

Earlier in this paper reference was made to Congressional interest in technology assessment. TA is a serious enterprise. It refers to the process of predicting the future consequences, especially the unintended consequences, of what we do with present technical knowledge. I believe it is urgent that professional practitioners whose business is primarily with disabled children, adopt a TA approach and contemplate more fully the public policy consequences of what others do with what we say we know: how ICD-based epidemiologic studies influence service appropriations; what parents do with labels; what Congressmen do with generalized aggregated statistics (*how many* gets to be so much more important than who!) [27] ; whether shibboleths about the importance of prevention forever put aside those for whom prevention did not work; what OMB does to the disabled when it manipulates chunks of money tagged as health versus other chunks tagged as social services; what economists do when they average per capita costs and apply the result to decision making about Medicare for the disabled.

Above all it is necessary to apply the constructs of TA to assess the manner in which *our concepts* about persons with developmental disabilities (based, as we hope they are, on the most valid as well as the most recent findings of the social, behavioral, and biologic sciences) are interpreted to makers of public policy and are reflected by them in the way they formulate that policy from day to day.

REFERENCES

1. Lemkau, P., Tietze, C., and Cooper, M.: Mental hygiene problems in an urban district. Mental Hygiene 26:100–119, 1941.

2. Roth, W. F., Jr., and Luton, F. H.: The mental health program in Tennessee. Am. J. Psychiatry 99:662–675, 1943.
3. Lemkau, P. V.: Epidemiological aspects. In DiMichael, S. G., and Slobody, L. (eds.): "The Evaluation and Treatment of the Mentally Retarded Child in Clinics." New York: National Association for Retarded Children, 1956.
4. Stein, Z. A., and Susser, M.: Changes over time in the incidence and prevalence of mental retardation. In Hellmuth, J. (ed.): "Exceptional Infant," New York: Brunner Mazel, 1971, vol. 2.
5. Stein, Z. A., and Susser, M.: Public health and mental retardation: New power and new problems. In Begab, M. J., and Richardson, S. A. (eds.): "The Mentally Retarded in Society: A Social Science Perspective." Baltimore: University Park Press, 1975.
6. Lapouse, R., and Weitzner, M.: Epidemiology. In Wortis, J. (ed.): "Mental Retardation – An Annual Review I." New York: Grune and Stratton, 1970.
7. Lemkau, P. V., and Imré, P. D.: Results of a field epidemiologic study. Am. J. Ment. Def. 73:858–863, 1969.
8. Imré, P. D.: Mental retardation in a Maryland county. In Monroe, R. R., Klee, G. D., and Brody, E. B. (eds.): "Psychiatric Epidemiology and Mental Health Planning." Psychiatric Research Report #22. Washington, D.C.: American Psychiatric Association, 1967.
9. Lemkau, P., Tietze, C., and Cooper, M.: Mental hygiene problems in an urban district. Mental Hygiene 26:275–288, 1942.
10. Lemkau, P., Tietze, C., and Cooper, M.: Mental hygiene problems in an urban district. Mental Hygiene 27:279–295, 1943.
11. Saenger, G.: "The Adjustment of Severely Retarded Adults in the Community." Albany: New York State Interdepartment Health Resources Board, 1957.
12. Kirk, S. A.: "Educating Exceptional Children." Boston: Houghton Mifflin, 1962.
13. Havemann, J.: Federalism report/state, local officials help write consolidation plans. National Journal 8:228–233, 1976.
14. Curlin, J. W.: Mutatis mutandis: Congress, science and law. (Editorial.) Science 190: 839, 1975.
15. Gurel, L.: The human side of evaluating human services programs. In Guttentag, M., and Struening, E. L. (eds.): "Handbook of Evaluation Research," Beverly Hills, Calif.: Sage, 1975, vol. 2, pp. 13–26.
16. Weiss, C. H.: Evaluation research in the political context. "Handbook of Evaluation Research," Ibid., vol. 1, pp. 11–28.
17. Hobbs, N.: "The Futures of Children." San Francisco: Jossey-Bass, 1975.
18. Boggs, E.: Issues in long term care for persons disabled early in life. In Knee, R., and McCuan, P. (eds.): "Human Factors in Long Term Health Care – Final Report of the Task Force." Washington, D.C. and Columbus, Ohio: National Conference on Social Welfare, 1975.
19. National Center for Social Statistics: Findings of the 1970 APTD Study Part I. Demographic and Program Characteristics, DHEW Pub. #(SRS) 73-03853. Washington, D.C.: Social and Rehabilitation Service, 1972.
20. Treitel, R.: Onset of disability. Reports from the Social Security Survey of the Disabled: 1966, #18. Washington, D. C.: Social Security Administration, Office of Research and Statistics, 1972.
21. Boggs, E. M.: Federal legislation 1966–71. In Wortis, J. (ed.): "Mental Retardation, An Annual Review IV." New York: Grune and Stratton, 1972.

22. Nielson, G., Collins, S., Meisel, J., et al: An intervention program for atypical infants. In Friedlander, B. Z., Sterritt, G. M., and Kirck, G. E. (eds.): "Exceptional Infant," New York: Brunner Mazel, 1975, vol. 3.
23. Conley, R. W.: An assessment of the economic and non-economic costs and benefits of mental retardation programs. In Cohen, J. S., Butter, I., Deline, S., and Nutter, R. (eds.): "Benefit-Cost Analysis for Mental Retardation Programs; Theoretical Considerations and a Model for Application." Ann Arbor, Mich.: Institute for the Study of Mental Retardation and Related Disabilities, 1971.
24. Bierman, J. M., Siegel, E., French, F. E., and Connor, A.: The community impact of handicaps of prenatal or natal origin. Public Health Rep. 78:839, 1963.
25. French, F. E., Connor, A., Bierman, J. M., et al: Congenital and acquired handicaps of ten-year-olds — Report of a follow-up study, Kuai, Hawaii. Am. J. Public Health 58:1388–1395, 1968.
26. Knee, R. (ed.): "Human Factors in Long-Term Care — Final Report of the Task Force." Washington, D.C. and Columbus, Ohio: National Conference on Social Welfare, 1975.
27. Gallagher, J. J., Forsythe, P., Ringelheim, D., and Weintraub, F. J.: Funding patterns and labeling. In Hobbs, N. (ed.): "Issues in the Classification of Children," San Francisco: Jossey-Bass, 1975, vol. II.

Adapting Environments for the Developmentally Disabled

Sandra C. Howell, PhD, MPH

Adopting the principle of normalization to the production or modification of environments for the developmentally disabled person will *not* necessarily promote optimum growth for these individuals. Normative environments are not now sufficiently sensitive to the functional capacities and developmental potentials of nondisabled persons. Therefore to mimic their inadequacies and call this therapeutic is to perform a major disservice to more vulnerable populations. This is not to say that the fervent efforts at personalizing residential institutions have been fruitless [1–3]. Reinforcements to emotional and social adjustment can support a positive learning experience. The learning experience, here considered to be the development of competence in environmental decision making, must still be scheduled.

The purpose of this presentation is to provide a set of recommended directions which those of you much more specialized in the field of developmental disability than I need to follow in order to be able to prepare an *e*ffective, as well as *a*ffective, environmental adaptation program.

I bring to this discussion a background in 3 increasingly interrelated fields: 1) public health, with particular emphasis upon out-of-hospital planning, especially for long-term care populations; 2) life-cycle developmental psychology (a recent attempt to see people as having growth and change potential from birth to death); and 3) environmental psychology, also a recently accredited field which explores the interactive effects of specific components of the human physicosocial environment with human behaviors [4, 5].

It was with considerable hesitation that I accepted the invitation to present this paper. I was sure those of you particularly involved with the mentally handicapped had it all together and that there would be little new that I could offer. I now find, with still some humility, that you may be going around in circles. A careful review of your most advanced literature dealing with alternative living environments strongly suggests that the systematic ways of behavioral science have been put aside in favor of polemics (albeit politically necessary) and insubstantial idealism [6–9].

The developmental potential of mentally handicapped children, with and without sensory-motor disabilities, is still not well documented. It would appear as if the specialists expected the leap from dependency to socialization to take place without the firm establishment of cognitive representations of environmental competencies. Child psychologists tend to concur that such a leap is not possible in normal development; it must be even more problematic for the handicapped. We have neglected to attend to the need for a functional analysis of settings and physical stimuli in order to understand the organization of responses which are seen in disabled children. How do specific characteristics of environments influence information processing or reinforce discrimination and generalization learning, and what properties of the environment elicit particular motor, verbal, and social responses in the mentally handicapped child [10]? While I can observe my young friend Rachel, at 18 months, visually and tactilly explore a knot in a pine cabinet and assume that this piece of incidental learning will be integrated as a part of normal cognitive development, I would not know what would be done with such environmental interactions by the mentally handicapped child. Some of the homelike personalizations of residential settings recommended for these children may, in fact, slow down or divert development rather than enhance their potential.

That we still base too much of our evaluation and environmental intervention strategies on the MA/CA ratio has not been critically reevaluated by most people in your field. The 8-year-old who functions at a 4-year-old level may be doing so because she/he is given 4-year-old environments or is offered problem solving situations that create noise in an information-processing system that cannot handle the speed or complexity (ambiguity) of stimulus inputs. Your literature does allude to stimulus deprivation and stimulus enhancement but rarely touches on the subjects of stimulus overload or stimulus appropriateness in relation to environmental adaptation issues. Discussion of the stimulus-deprived environments of institutions has been rampant in the retarded field. It is interesting to note that research suggests that early, enriched environments more positively affect mentally incapacitated and that brighter individuals, more than duller, are affected by deprivation [11]. In other words, we might argue that the sooner a systematic program of environmental stimulation is provided to the developmentally disabled the better the promise of progress in learning. The 8-year-old has 4 years of environmental interactions over the 4-year-old, no matter what the level of mental handicap. The reinforcing properties of those environments and their spatial components, in terms of enhancement or retardation of responses, have yet to be specified in scientific terms.

I notice in the literature that attempts are being made to evolve criterion-referenced tests or inventories of individual competencies. Such evaluation protocols, which use the individual's functional capacities as his/her own base line and change measure, promise to provide superior material on which to plan educational and environmental interventions. The weaknesses of such systems, as their authors acknowledge, lie in the still subjective quality of the entries (inter-rater reliability has not been well controlled). In addition, such instruments as the Progress Assessment Chart (PAC) still are overly targeted to "social competence" without first breaking down the possible sensory-motor and cognitive skills that require parallel or even preliminary mastery [1].

My role as a consultant psychologist to the architecture profession has increasingly turned to assisting in the translation of behavioral goals for the purpose of specifying recommended elements of a design program. There are, both in Europe and America, a few examples of such programming efforts. I site particularly the efforts of Bayes and Francklin [12] and Reeves [13]. In the latter case, a set of design patterns is actually formatted in anticipation of systematic evaluation of user impact.

Pattern 1.4: Neighborhood Organization and Paths

It is easy to accept that institutional places are dull and confusing and uncomprehensible; that is the way they always have been. But what goes unseen is how this limited environment pushes residents towards the very sort of withdrawal that may have gotten them there in the first place. Forced associations and limited options make destructive behavior, such as fighting, more likely. People also act more afraid and withdrawn if the place is disorienting.

    Understimulation
    Options/Choice
    Focus/Comprehension

What follows are specific recommendations for designating, via consistent form, color or materials, directions, spaces and objects.

Pattern 3.12: Lighting Which Defines Space and Activity

How lighting is arranged and how it is controlled can say a great deal about what kind of place you are in. Is it a home that belongs to somebody? What does the lighting say about those who use the space? Are they important individuals or just part of a large mass? Does anyone care about making sure the lights are turned off when they're not being used? Or do rows and rows of fixtures stay on until some "official" person comes along to shut them off?

      Identify/Choice
      Responsiveness
      Focus/Stimulation
      Spirit/Warmth

Still these and less ambitious environmental prescriptions do not provide clear connections between developmental goals that can be specifically associated with classifiable functional disabilities. I am referring here particularly to cognitive and sensory-perceptual development, since it appears that personal-social development goals are, in fact, being sensitively considered by the *avant garde* in your field [14, 15].

Without regard for the fine accuracy of the proposed elements, consider a format such as described in Table 1 as potentially very valuable to innovative and experimental architecture for the mentally handicapped.

By following a programming format such as this, an institution, school or residence may be better able to support, environmentally, the therapeutic goals of parents, teachers and physicians. A fourth column would be added to this table in planning a specific environment that would recommend solutions, *in design*

TABLE 1. Environmental Programming Process

Developmental status (Disability characteristics at baseline)	Developmental goal	Design program elements
See and refine evaluation methods such as Gunzburgs' PAC.	Discrimination learning	Clearly differentiated spaces and objects. Consistent signs.
	Generalization of responses	Redundant cues. Varieties of similar-use spaces and objects.
	Spatial orientation	Consistent directional language. Differential space specification.
	Sensory-motor problem solving	Alternative repetitive spatial, textural, and structural components.
	Stimulation: exploration and curiosity	Manipulable objects, spaces, and fixtures.
	Depth perception	Clean definition of edges, ridges, steps. Contrasts.
	Visual and auditory tracking	Correlation of color cues with goal; visual localization of sounds.

terms, appropriate for a particular room, building, or detail. Scientific method involves specifying all stimulus inputs and classifying them in some appropriate way. Home (family) environments may have to be modified in "unhomelike" ways to maximize opportunities of the mentally handicapped child to learn, or to reinforce expert school environments in key ways at key development points.

CAN ENVIRONMENTAL COMPONENTS BE SPECIFIED?

If developmental goals are clearly delineated, environmental interventions which may or may not contribute to development and behavior change ought to be able also to be specified. The problems of designing living laboratories (in homes or institutional facilities) center around holding extraneous social-environmental variables constant while changing single or only a few components. Usually when design adaptations are made, too many new environmental qualities are simultaneously introduced. Of course, an ideal principle would be to add variables (interventions) one at a time so that their interactive effects can be measured.

CAN THE IMPACT OF ENVIRONMENTAL COMPONENTS BE MEASURED?

Behavior change is the core measure in psychology. In order to assess a change in behavior, an initial state has to be recorded. In the case of environmental interventions, this initial state of *person-function must relate to the context*, or environmental inputs, at the time of the first evaluation. Intervening variables between pre- and postmeasures must also be specified. For example, in the case of measuring the effects of single- vs two-person bedrooms, a change in the composition of staff, living group members, or other spatial modifications could distort the impact measure [1, 13, 16, 17].

In Figure 1 some general models for environmental intervention research and practice are outlined which perhaps need to be restated here because of the tendency still to think that any home setting is better than any institutional setting.

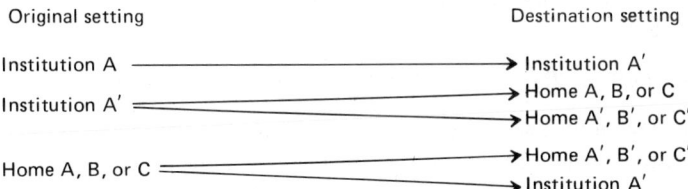

Fig. 1. Alternative research models. Where A, B, or C = environmentally *un*controlled settings; A', B', or C' = environmentally controlled settings. Both original and destination settings need to be subjected to specific environmental and individual functional assessments.

What must be remembered is that the current and not too adequate research model is from Institution A ⟶ Home A, B — that is, from a traditional, dormitory-hospital setting to a parental or foster home of an unspecified, but more intimate, character.

TOWARD A RADICAL REINTERPRETATION

Developing a position on environment and human behavior would be no fun without some radical speculation. I want to call your attention to research on perception conducted with people whose daily learning experiences were *not* transferrable to 2-dimensional test protocols [18, 19]. Is it possible that the integration and organization of sensory-motor experiences for use by some segments of the mentally handicapped child population could be considered as unsocialized to our cognitive culture? That is to say, depth, edges, localization of points and sounds in space are taken in very pragmatically in terms of immediate use. If this is so, all other things being equal (particularly the control of ambiguity), such a person would not respond well to most standardized aural-spatial tests *until taught the translation!*

The implications of this type of rethinking are vast. While we are attempting to normalize the environment and its stimulus configurations and assist the handicapped to become socialized in their learning experiences, their cognitive proclivities may be "if it feels good, or works, do it!" Of course this is an oversimplified analogy, but I sense in the literature a rigidity about response appropriateness and sequential learning that may be severely biased by what we now measure as normal development for children in Western industrialized society. I charge you also to look to underachieving bright children from a perspective other than purely psychoanalytic. Some of them, too, are "marching to a different drummer" with regard to living/learning environments. I am not at all sure but that some proportion of dyslectic children perceive the symbolic and reactive world as truly disassociated from the English language (and its bizarre spelling), and this may be explained ultimately, in terms of an alternative cognitive structure. The so-called hyperactive child forced to sit in a constant spatial matrix may be seeking cognitive inputs which the environment of the schoolroom disallows.

ADAPTING ENVIRONMENTS, WHAT IS POSSIBLE NOW?

The search for better methods of evaluating the environmental capacities of the mentally handicapped and for researching specific environmental therapies is a long-term goal. Like the overgrieving widower who was reassured he would find a new mate we must ask, "But what will I do tonite, Rabbi?"

1) Continue efforts to personalize residential settings. Walls that can take pictures and mirrors; window sills and open shelves that can take plants, books, treasured toys.

2) Develop a sense of appropriate human scale for living centers. Break up large rooms into focal areas. Use differential lighting to support this variety. Selectively lower high ceilings. Modify or eliminate long corridors with undifferentiated doors going off on both sides.

3) Provide clearer markings within residential and nonresidential buildings to orient people of all ages to where they are, where they want to go, and how to get there and back.

4) Develop residential spaces that permit choice in social interaction, from privacy through dyad to small group. Attend to acoustic management of these spaces. Some activities should communicate that life is going on, others require damping down; guided selection of interior surface materials will provide this distinction.

5) Attend to the positive *and negative* affects of circulation paths through residential settings. While they serve to encourage informal social interaction, they can also interrupt or distract attention and concentration. Walk through settings and observe others doing so, to determine where circulation should be rerouted by erection of dividers.

6) Call attention, by location and accentuation, to competence-developing building hardware and fixtures. Clearly specify light switches, heat controls, storage areas, and where possible, provide a variety of hardware types to facilitate learning that windows, doors, and faucets come in a variety of materials and shapes.

7) Eliminate architectural barriers that could result in accidents or reduce opportunity for realizing success in sensory-motor and problem-solving activities [20]; for example, a) stairs of inconsistent riser height and without handsized railings; b) stoves with poorly marked dials located behind the burners.

8) Provide particular rooms with enough space to facilitate teaching of daily living and social competencies, eg bathrooms which allow a second person to teach personal hygiene, kitchens which permit 3–4-person activities related to food preparation; bedrooms that allow 2–3-person play or talk groups [21].

9) Develop in-service and parent education programs in environmental management, then reinforce these in relation to the particular needs of the individual child and care giver.

10) Stay close to your architect, interior designer, and contractors and monitor *every* decision that is made in relation to the behavioral objectives you have for your residents. Think more than twice about gimicky decorating tricks in terms of possible disorienting, ambiguous, or frightening effects.

Finally, communicate, in writing, your professional experiences and observations with regard to environmental manipulations. Describe what you did, for what anticipated behavioral objective to work and for what kind of persons

For our part, as researchers, we will try to do the same for you: translate our too often garbage language into usable "show and tell" verse [22].

REFERENCES

1. Gunzburg, H. C., and Gunzburg, A. L.: "Mental Handicap and Physical Environment." Baltimore: The Williams and Wilkins Co., 1973.
2. Gruenwald, K.: "The Guiding Environment: The Dynamics of Residential Living." U.S. Department of HEW, SRS.
3. Sarason, S. B.: "The Creation of New Settings and Future Societies." San Francisco: Jossey-Bass, 1972.
4. Craik, K.: Environmental psychology. In Newcomb, T. (ed.): "New Directions in Psychology," New York: Holt, Rinehart & Winston, 1970, vol. 4, pp. 1–121.
5. Moos, R. H.: "Evaluating Treatment Environments: A Social Ecological Approach." New York: John Wiley & Sons, 1974.
6. Cherington, C., and Dybwad, G.: "New Neighbors: The Retarded Citizen in Quest of a Home." President's Committee on Mental Retardation, 1974.
7. Ganges, A. G.: "New Environments for Retarded People." DHEW publication # (OHD) 75-21009, President's Committee on Mental Retardation. (Architectural exhibits from 4th World Congress, 1972.)
8. Dickman, I. R.: "No Place Like Home: Alternative Living Arrangements for Teenagers and Adults With Cerebral Palsy." New York: United Cerebral Palsy Associations, Inc., 1975. Monograph.
9. Elliott, J., and Bayes, K.: "Room for Improvement a Better Environment for the Mentally Handicapped." King Edward's Hospital Fund for London, 1972.
10. Bijou, S. W.: Development in the preschool years: A functional analysis. Am. Psychologist 829–837, 1975.
11. Thompson, W. R. and Schaefer, T.: Early environment stimulation. In Fiske, D. W., and Maddi, S. R. (eds.): "Functions of Varied Experience." Homewood, Illinois: Dorsey Press, 1961, Ch. 4.
12. Bayes, K., and Francklin, S.: The therapeutic environment. King Edwards Hospital Fund for London, 1973. (Monograph.)
13. Reeves, R.: "Handbook/Changing Places and Settings." Architecture: Research Construction (ARC), Cleveland, Ohio, 1975.
14. Centre on Environment for the Handicapped: "Design for Mentally Handicapped People." Bibliography/Information Sheet. London: November 1972. (Mimeograph.)
15. Committee on Architectural Planning of the International League of Societies for the Mentally Handicapped. Newsletter 3, October 1972.
16. Wolfe, M.: Room size, group size and density: Behavior patterns in a children's psychiatric facility. Environment and Behavior 7:199–224, 1975.
17. Paluck, R. J., and Esser, A. H.: Territorial behavior as an indicator of changes in clinical behavioral condition of severely retarded boys. Am. J. Ment. Defic. 76:284–290, 1971.
18. Segall, M. H., Campbell, D. T., and Herskovity, M. J.: "The Influence of Culture on Visual Perception." New York: Bobbs-Merril, 1966.
19. Deregowski, J. R.: Pictorial perception and culture. Sci. Am. 5:82–88, 1972.
20. Steinfeld, E.: "Interim Report: Barrier-Free Access to the Man-Made Environment." Washington, D. C.: Dept. Housing and Urban Development. October 1975.
21. Reizenstein, J., and McBride, W.: Design for Normalization: A Social-Environmental Evaluation of a Community for Retarded Adults. Journal of Architectural Research, 1976. (Submitted for publication.)
22. Willems, E. P.: "Place and Motivation: Independence and Complexity in Patient Behavior." Proceedings of Environment-Design Research Assoc. 1:4–1–1, 4–3–8, 1972.

Developmental Disabilities: Educating the Public

Lowell S. Levin, EdD, MPH

To begin with a personal disclaimer is in order. My health education experience in practice and research has never focused on any of the conditions clustered under the rubric of "developmental disabilities." Indeed, I was not even sure of this fact until an informal survey of laws, literature, and colleagues formed a body of opinion on the scope of the referent conditions. And that body of opinion is by no means a consensus, because, as I discovered, the notion of developmental disability, unlike disease classifications, appears to have emerged out of a confluence of social and political strategies to a much greater degree than out of commonalities in etiology, symptoms, or treatment. It became absolutely clear that the referent disease state(s) was an almost irrelevant criterion for inclusion in contrast to the criterion of the illness state — the individual's and society's response to disease or anomalies which originate at birth or in childhood. Within this domain, the central concerns are largely victim centered, eg physical/emotional disability limitation with special emphasis on improving, coping, or adaptive behavior or concerns of modifying the behavior of therapists, teachers, and families of the developmentally disabled. This is not to say that matters of public values and attitudes regarding the developmentally disabled have been unappreciated by scholars or practitioners, but by and large undertakings directed at the public's perspective and performance are scarce indeed. A relatively fruitless review of this aspect of developmental disability control, coupled with the intriguing challenge of illness education in contrast to disease education, emboldens me to test some ideas regarding the problem of public education on developmental disabilities and some alternatives in change.

The course of ideas to be charted demands first of all some rather definite statements with regard to health education and the assumptions and values it represents. There are, of course, divergent views on this, so it may be helpful to know the nature of my biases. My construction of health education rests on certain beliefs and nonbeliefs about health and disease and the role of education in our society. These notions can be summarized briefly.

1) With regard to health and disease: I believe that the separation of these concepts — particularly the radical differentiation of them as polar values — is at best dysfunctional and at worst a source of socially induced iatrogenesis. A pristine concept of health derives from a devil theory of disease and suggests the religious origins of the disease professions. The concept of disease as social deviance rooted in such a transcendent nomism can lead only to intractable and intransigent adherence to stereotypic behavior and its consequences, eg fear, stigma, guilt, and avoidance. Yet the devil theory of disease is commonplace and unchallenged. Indeed, as Margaret Mead pointed out, such values have been institutionalized in our various religious wars, or crusades, against disease. The militancy of our efforts to stamp out disease (or presumably the final insult, death) simply reinforce the popular belief in the devil theory. The irony is manifest. I would argue for a perspective on health and disease which champions neither but, rather, establishes the relationship of the human condition to ignorance of sources of risk, ignorance of decision-making strategies, and ignorance of personal and social options to achieve fulfillment.

2) With regard to education in our society: Education is a process of self-actualization. The Brazilian educational philosopher, Paolo Freire, expressed it this way:

> I cannot think *for others* or *without others*, nor can others think *for me*. Even if the people's thinking is superstitious or naive, it is only as they rethink their assumptions in action that they can change. Producing and acting upon their own ideas — not consuming those of others — must constitute that process [1].

Such a view of education implies an emphasis on learning skills of inquiry and criticism rather than on the assimilation of the educator's values and ritual adaptation to norms. What is at stake here is the integrity of the individual as a decision-making resource in social change. To implement this educational strategy will require more than cosmetic adjustments in the style of educators; it will require abandonment of behavior-modification enterprises which do not contribute to (indeed bypass) the development of skills central to effective self-determinism. It is in this cause that education in health can best serve to reduce not disease and not necessarily the illness associated with it but the larger debilitating consequences of public ignorance — dependency and its sequel, social control. Surely we are witness now to the negative benefits of an educational approach which has failed to acknowledge, much less nurture, people's appreciation for the utility of insight, their competence to critically assess information, their ability to rationally undertake personal and social decision making, and their confidence to undertake effective action as they see it.

With these views set out as my frame of educational reference, I now want to turn to the specific consideration of development disabilities and public education about them. It is clear from commentaries heard here and elsewhere that there exists a wide range of public prejudice with regard to handicaps and health deviance in general and that these prejudices work in subtle, and not so subtle, ways to shut down or severely limit opportunities for the full expression of human worth be it in terms of physical and emotional habilitation, employment, or the general civil and social functions of children and adults. When such prejudice occurs within the various social support systems — medicine, education, and the law — specific remedies are attempted or suggested. And given adequate financial, technical, and ethical resources, there is at least a plausible strategy available to pursue changes in service procedures, care-giver behavior (professional or parental), and, in theory at least, attitudes associated with the performance of service. The system itself has at least access to the system — a known entity whose identity and legitimacy are based on defined social contracts or fiduciary relationships. We know the nature of the care-giver process: the recruitment of individuals into the provider system; the content, structure, and process of their professionalization; the milieu of their work place; the location, charter, and dimensions of community services; and the myriad of other attributes of the care system both real and potential. We can appreciate the options in placing our own house in order — to reform the system. We have at hand (and are always seeking more) ways of enforcement of performance standards through personnel screening, curriculum reform, audit systems, and public accountability procedures, including advocacy programs and legal devices to protect clients from abuse. It is no surprise, therefore, to find that most of our efforts to improve the prejudicial state of affairs for the developmentally disabled appear to have been concentrated on that part of the social system over which we have most control, the disabled themselves and the support system that serves them.

But in the public domain of stigma and prejudice we appear to have no apparent handle on intervention or enforcement. The public behavior with regard to the developmentally disabled is governed by values and beliefs, by expectations and rewards, by knowledge and skills which are largely the product of socialization, pervasive, diverse, and often even impossible to define. This lack of systems control over society-at-large has caused efforts at public attitude change to be limited to *pro forma* media appeals and pamphleteering which have had little demonstrable impact. By and large we have concluded, on the one hand, that the public is subject to highly competitive demands and is reluctant to share finite social goods, that the pressure for peer acceptance depresses tolerance for deviance, and that latent public guilt results in massive denial of personal responsibility. We do discern, on the other hand, that not all categories of disability are subject to the same level of diffidence or rejection. John Kershaw [2] provides us with a cogent review of variations in public attitudes as they relate to the war disabled, the blind, the deaf, the epileptic, the physically deformed, the mentally retarded, and the spastic. It is clear that public attitudes and behavior toward the disabled are not a monolith and may indeed, as Kershaw points out, reflect in their variation significant differences in the public's view of their collective responsibility for the cause of the disability (as in the case of the disabled veteran) or in the public's ability to easily imagine and appreciate the nature of the disability (as in blindness).

There appear to be 2 concerns about public attitudes and behavior with regard to the developmentally disabled — namely, increasing public support for additional and more effective professional services to the disabled and improving public acceptance of the disabled in the mainstream of society. There can be no doubt of the extraordinary level of public initiative in pressing for increases in, and the rationality of, professional resources to benefit the developmentally disabled. The Developmental Disabilities Services and Facilities Construction Act (Public Law 91-517) and its Title II amendment the Developmentally Disabled Assistance and Bill of Rights Act of 1974 are testimony to the persistence and assiduity of mobilized public action, more particularly the coalition of individuals with practical and immediate concerns for the care or welfare of the disabled and voluntary associations with compatible categoric interests. In effect, legislation on behalf of the developmentally disabled is the result of a form of class action to correct service deficiencies or inequities in extant services. And although this process may be circumspect in its popular base, namely, limited to those with special interest in disabilities, it surely reflects a broader shift in the public response to social inequities in general, eg minorities, women, homosexuals. So there is a tide of activism, which suggests a steady continuation of positive results, temporary retrenchments notwithstanding.

But there is another aspect to the reforms we have seen regarding increased access and improved services, an aspect which may have profound effects on the other side of the public behavior equation, that is, the improvement of public acceptance of the developmentally disabled into the social mainstream. The pursuit of reforms in the health and educational systems, as it represents the present thrust of social action, assumes that the solutions to the problems at issue lie within those systems. While there is little doubt that medical and educational systems have certainly contributed, evidence of profound solutions is less clear. Indeed, if one examines the institutional contexts in which alleged benefits are provided, one must take into account the deficit of iatrogenesis contributed by those environments. Now, no reasonable argument can be made for the immediate abandonment of technical/social support systems for the disabled, but by the same token there must be in place the realization of 1) the limits of this technology in terms of quality, cost, and availability; 2) its negative side effects (or inappropriateness when dealing with the political and social aspects of disability); and 3) the distortion it precipitates (or reinforces) in obfuscating the potential for public, nonprofessional responsibility [3]. By directing our social muscle at systems reform, we have created the easy illusion that that is where the action is, and society has risen to this bait enticed by the simplicity of the solution as advertised. It is little wonder that the general state of the public mind, while liberalized in terms of its acceptance of a more egalitarian view of access to care and institutional reform, has, if anything, become less inclined (and may perceive itself as less able) to undertake more self-directed responsibility not only for the care of the developmentally disabled but for their social growth as well. And it is this latter goal which seems to be the ultimate achievement and the least likely to be advanced through any system of care which is a surrogate for society-at-large.

Given that we can assume a nonsystem, nonprofessional model of "intervention" in the care and growth of the developmentally disabled as necessary (for purposes of universal access), as rational (based on the largely sociopolitical nature of the problem), and as desirable (in terms of impact on the general growth of social competence in society), what strategy(ies) is appropriate to implement such a model?

I suggest an essentially educational approach which would include several objectives or foci which interrelate in time and interact in impact. The strategy certainly would not be exclusive of nor deny the benefits of continuing political and legal efforts to rectify civil inequities, nor would it assume a reduced support for research in primary prevention, nor should it demand total commitment in the face of unproved results. It should be undertaken in the spirit of experimentation and innovation in an effort to test the proposition that the ideal is to achieve a caring environment in society as the primary resource with institutionalized support systems (clinics, schools) as secondary resources. This would involve the creation — and in some instances the re-creation — of sensitivities, perspectives, and skills which constitute a social model of activity and foster a public alert to its potential to serve itself and to know how and what and when to use professional resources. This is clearly a reductionist view which holds that professional intervention is in its ultimate effect essentially conservative and self-preservative creating public responsiveness, and diluting the genuine and specific contribution of professional resources.

Public education of children offers an accessible and nearly universal leverage point for change. We can begin by an approach to health education which strengthens skills of observation and inquiry using epidemiology as the organizing educational framework. Children can be given an opportunity to sense themselves as a legitimate resource of ideas, beliefs, and values associated with disease and disability through exercises which allow an open and nondirective production of views regarding causation; variations in risk; treatment and prognosis; and psychologic, social, political, and economic factors as interactive (complicit) and consequential. It should become evident and credible to students that definitions, perspectives, and interventions in health are fundamentally cultural and that the professional system in response is merely an institutionalization of some of these cultural values. Such a tiny point, and yet it is a concept whose appreciation can begin to dissolve the myth of the health-disease dichotomy and establish the nature of the individual's role in causation and control.

The second educational step involves the conversion of beliefs into hypotheses and procedures to test them within the context of the students' own community. This process should contribute to a shattering of monolithic stereotypes and the commensurate emergence of, in the case of disability, the normalization of deviance. It also should contribute to a sense of the range of human behaviors which are not affected by a particular disability, thereby diminishing the disability stereotype of diffuse impairment.

The capstone of this approach must be the opportunity for students to draw conclusions regarding personal behavior in terms of dealing with their own and others' disabilities — their own in the sense of compensatory and coping behavior and with regard to others in the sense of their views on community action, services, and legislation. This aspect of the process is crucial in the development of high quality decision-making skills and, therefore, must conform to rigorous procedures of data analysis and assessment. This means that teachers must be able to forego the temptation to reward or punish decisions which may or may not conform to their criteria. The key outcome here is to give students confidence in their obligations and rights in decision making as well as confidence in their method of self-determination.

Corollary to the above approach to demystification of health, disease, disability, and their sequelae and to the strengthening of the lay role in decision making, we must consider ways of building a medical self-care capability in the lay component of the consumer-provider dyad. Self-care education is concerned with building personal health skills which cover the spectrum of behaviors related to health promotion, diagnosis, and treatment of disease or injury, rehabilitation, and disability limitation. Competence within each of these areas would include functions supplementary, substitutionary, and additive to the traditional professional care domain of service. Thus defined, self-care must be considered an integral part of the health care system — indeed the largest component considering the potential contributions of 200 plus million self-care competent lay persons. The theoretic, technical, economic, and social rationales for self-care are the subject of several recent and forthcoming international and national conferences which have addressed the issue of the limits of medicine — and public health for that matter — in really improving the health of populations [4]. In addition, self-care is being popularized through a vast array of advisories, manuals, lay-oriented algorithms and protocols, and encyclopedias [5]. Groups with special self-care interests have grown exponentially, stimulated by the pioneering efforts of the women's movement. Presently there are purposeful educational programs in self-care for women, residents of medically underserved areas, and ordinary citizens who want to gain more control over their personal health care [6]. With regard to children, there is a beginning interest in designing an educational approach which will help children learn how to take the initiative in health decision making. The work of Mary Ann Lewis at UCLA is noteworthy in this regard [7]. Lewis recast the decision-making relationship between the student and school nurse. Students were given the responsibility to determine their illness status and take the initiative in deciding on the treatment plan. The nurse reinforced this process by suggesting the treatment options available and supporting the students' decision.

The strengthening of lay competence in decision making and the strengthening of their confidence in primary self-care competence certainly must be expected to create a psychologic environment conducive to significant changes in public perspectives on developmental disability and its collective behavioral response. This assertion, or hypothesis, is grounded on the belief that the barriers to effective public performance in the matter of developmental disabilities are not specific to the concept of disability itself but are more generally related to the diffuse misconceptions held regarding the health-disease model and the taboos associated with it. In my view, it will be a far more fruitful undertaking to encourage the growth of a new public perspective on health, and individual potential in health, than to slug away at the constantly regenerative responses of stigma, stereotyping, and avoidance. We need not abandon — nor should we — educational efforts to treat one or another surface aspect of the problem (such as sensitization workshops) [8], but surely these activities must be seen as palliative and difficult to apply on a mass scale.

How realistic is the suggestion that we pursue a developmentally oriented educational approach in contrast to behavior-modification strategies of the usual sort based on prejudged professional outcome criteria? The question has several dimensions — time, cost, cost-effectiveness, resources availability, philosophic and cultural fit, technical displacements, side effects (educational iatrogenesis), and, of course, political reverberations in the care-giver industries. I do not know the answer, except to be reasonably sure that we would be facing a 25–30-year process before the benefit ratios would become substantially favorable. And that may be a conservative estimate, given the Swedish government's expectation of the same time frame to achieve significant changes in smoking behavior through considerably more directive means. Passivity, fear and avoidance, and stereotyping behavior have become virtual cultural artifacts, as has the dependency-producing orientation of the helping professions which inadvertently, perhaps, has contributed so much to these mental sets. It may, indeed, be more difficult to turn around the professions than the public itself! In any case, we have a long haul ahead of us. An ameliorating factor with regard to time, however, may be that the process of improving decision making and lay care-giving skills represents a process, in part at least, of flowing with the current of change in society's general interest in achieving more self-control, reducing anomie, and challenging authoritarian values whether they are political or medical. Certainly the growing demand for popular access to certain skills heretofore solely in the professional domain is the basis for some optimism. In effect what is being proposed is more on the order of accelerated evolution than revolution.

At the moment we have the conceptual elements of an educational approach requiring test *in situ* within a community or communities willing to undertake an educational strategy of the self-determining type described earlier. The health professions serving those communities, the teachers, and the children, parents, and adults involved must be participants in the planning of an on-going program. A concerted, longitudinal design is clearly as requisite in health behavior research as it is in heart disease. The newly designated Health Service areas may offer ideal experimental environments for such undertakings, on the basis that the HSA represents an effective opportunity for coordinate and integrated planning. The health education inputs would be derived from the general conceptual model-changing perspectives on health and disease and from strengthening individual competence and initiatives in health behavior. Considerable lattitude for methodologic and evaluative strategies would be encouraged and agreed as they are compatible with the overall conceptual criteria, eg stimulate the learner to produce and act upon his or her own ideas, contribute to a rational technique of health decision making, normalize the notions of health initiatives, contribute skills of self-competence in health care, establish a sense of the social model in health, and foster more precise but more limited professional intervention in the health-care process.

The thesis of this paper is that significant changes in public behavior regarding the developmentally disabled can only occur through more fundamental shifts in the public's orientation toward themselves as the universal and primary resource in health and as secure and confident in that role. The subsequent demystification of health, disease, and disability should result in a corollary dissolution of the prejudicial behavior toward the developmentally disabled. Mainstreaming the developmentally disabled is one useful and necessary approach, but at the same time we must begin to broaden and deepen the perspective and the competence of the mainstream itself to ensure that we are not merely substituting tolerance and benevolence for the goal of a mature and interdependent society.

REFERENCES

1. Freire, P.: "Pedagogy of the Oppressed." New York: The Seabury Press, 1974, p. 100.
2. Kershaw, J. D.: "Handicapped Children." London: William Heinemann Medical Books, Ltd., 1973, pp. 12–19.
3. For a discussion of the limits and hazards of the professional care system see: McKnight, J.: The medicalization of politics. Paper presented at a conference on "The Limits of Medicine," Davos, Switzerland, March 1975. (Mimeograph.) (Available from the author, Center for Urban Affairs, Northwestern University, Evanston, Ill.)
4. Levin, L. S., Katz, A. H., and Holst, E.: "Self-Care; Changing Roles of the Individual in Health Services." New York: Neale Watson Academic Publications, Inc., 1976. (In preparation.)
5. Levin, L. S.: Self-care in health: Selected annotated bibliography. (Mimeograph.) (Available from the author, Yale University School of Medicine, Department of Epidemiology and Public Health, 60 College Street, New Haven, Conn.)
6. Sehnert, K. W., and Nocerino, J. T.: Course guide for the activated patient. A consumer-oriented program in preventive medicine and self-help medicine. Georgetown University School of Medicine, Department of Community Medicine and International Health, Washington, D.C. (Mimeograph.)
7. Lewis, M. A.: Child-initiated care. Am. J. Nurs. 74:652–655, 1974.
8. Ballou, B., and Todd, T. W.: Understanding developmental disabilities, A "sensitization" workshop program. Child. Today 2(5):28–29, 1973.

Medical Ecology: The Epidemiology of Handicap

Leon Eisenberg, MD

This Symposium in honor of Paul Lemkau expresses the debt of each of the speakers to Professor Lemkau as teacher, as colleague and as friend; and it also reflects the importance, for the future of public health, of his contribution in bringing the insights of epidemiology to bear on psychiatric problems as prototypes of chronic disease. Unless one attempts to assess the burden to the community in terms of disability as well as death represented by the ills that plague mankind, one has no meaningful guidelines for the setting of priorities or for the evaluation of outcomes. Norman Sartorius, the Chief of the Office of Mental Health of the World Health Organization, wanted to be sure that I called attention to Paul's contributions on the international scene. That there is a tradition of social psychiatric investigation in Yugoslavia is due primarily to the efforts of Professor Lemkau, beginning in the postwar period and continuing to the present.

It is manifestly impossible to comment in detail on each of the chapters included in this volume. Rather, I shall use some of the presentations as a taking-off point for discussion of some of the major themes that recur in the study of developmental disabilities.

Dr. Miller provided a lucid account of the history of the evolution of the British Columbia Case Register. It is clear that progress in designing and in evaluating services is impossible without knowledge of the size and extent of the health problem, its distribution in the community, the longitudinal course of illness (that is, its natural history) and the long-term consequences of the services that have been provided. In pursuit of this theme, I propose to set before you three complex case illustrations of the perspective provided by an epidemiologic frame which considerably alter the conclusions one might have come to from a purely clinical analysis.

First, both Dr. Anderson and Dr. Duff have already discussed some issues pertinent to spina bifida. What merits emphasis is the increasing burden of chronic illness and handicap that results from the very virtuosity of modern medicine. We now succeed in saving infants who once would have died. According to Laurence [1], present methods of care have increased the survivorship of such infants from 17% 20 years ago to 50% in the present decade. This is a tribute to neurosurgical skill. But before we celebrate this outcome, it should be noted that the number of functional survivors out of each birth cohort of 100 has increased from 8 to 15 whereas the number of paralyzed, doubly incontinent and severely defective children has increased from 5 to 27. Thus, for each additional 7 children with spina bifida to whom we are now able to offer a relatively normal life, we produce more than 20 additional severely disabled survivors. If we compute the average expectancy for this defect and apply the British data to the somewhat more than 3,000,000 live births in the United States, each year we are committing some 1,700 additional families to the painful experience of living with, or placing out, a severely handicapped child. This brings into focus the ethical questions so clearly outlined by Dr. Duff. The necessity to make the decision for or against surgery after birth is an agonizing one.

When other instances of spinal or cranial dysraphism are known to have occurred in a family, amniocentesis of the pregnant woman can ascertain elevated levels of alpha fetoprotein as a basis for therapeutic abortion. Unfortunately, this preventive measure is only applicable to that minority of cases with a family history. Even here we face ethical issues that trouble some. They may object to terming therapeutic abortion "preventive medicine." It has been argued that if we permit an unborn life to be terminated, we are on the slippery slope that will inevitably lead to enforced euthanasia for undesirables. This argument, if consistently applied, will bar contraception by any method as the first misstep on the road to perdition. In my view, the domino theory of the sequential collapse of moral values fiercely misrepresents the actuality of social behavior. Since the Supreme Court decision, legal abortions have occurred on a wide scale without any move to sanction the killing of live-born children. Indeed, the legislated sanctimoniousness that was law in the United States until that decision led directly to substantial death and disability from clandestine abortions for disadvantaged women. Advocates in behalf of the products of conception while they are in utero have little to say about the rights of children once they are born. Consider the iniquity of the conviction of Dr. Edelin for aborting a black fetus who, had he survived to ride a bus in Boston, might well have been stoned by those who "defend" fetal rights.

Let me turn to a second example: the formidable problem of evaluating the efficacy of the medical treatment of syphilis in the absence of knowledge of the distribution or course of the disease. As McDermott [2] has pointed out, syphilis was regarded as an ominous disorder by both patient and physician well into the 1950s. It was only 20 years ago that a Norwegian study revealed that the threat, though hardly trivial, was much less severe than had been taken to be the case. Gjsetland was able to show that if one acquired syphilis and received no treatment, the chance of developing a serious late form of the disease was only 15 in 100. This discovery came about only because of the availability of systematic records kept by a physician a half century earlier. Boeck, a physician in Oslo, disbelieved the conventional medical wisdom that mercury was an effective means of treating syphilis. Consequently, during the period 1890 to 1910, he kept all of the patients he diagnosed with early syphilis in Oslo as hospital inpatients until the surface lesions had healed. During the 1940s, Gjestland was able to trace most of Boeck's patients who had not been treated. By examining most of the survivors and obtaining reliable information about those who had died, he was able to reconstruct the natural history of the disease.

The case of syphilis is instructive as an indication of the dilemmas we face today in evaluating other chronic diseases with a long-term course. We can hardly repeat the experiment (how can we deny "treatment" that is thought to be effective in the absence of a better alternative?). Social policy decisions cannot be postponed for a half century while data are accumulated. Yet, in the absence of systematic data, we face a very real probability of introducing treatments that may carry as much or even more hazard as the disease.

My third example is one that stresses the urgent necessity of measuring the impact of medical and social interventions on human ecology; that is, on man *and* his environment. Just how complex these interrelations are can be illustrated by the effects of control measures for African trypanosomiasis [3]. African sleeping sickness of man and nagana of cattle are both caused by trypanosomes transmitted by the tsetse fly. In the Sahel desert margin, successful chemoprophylaxis against nagana resulted in a sizable increase in the cattle population. This, in turn, led to overgrazing of areas of grassland barely able to support the smaller herds that had existed in the past. So extensive has this overgrazing become that it has actually altered the reflectivity of the earth to the sun's light. Surface reflectivity is an important factor in determining patterns of rainfall. All other conditions being constant, high reflectivity (which characterizes a desert surface) can reduce rainfall by as much as 50% to 70%. Thus, the following train of events contributed to the Sahel drought and the tragedy of human starvation: more effective trypanosomiasis control led to larger herds of cattle and greater ability of their herders to spread them over wider zones; the increased number of cattle resulted in severe overgrazing of grassland; this then increased the reflectivity of the surface and led to smaller rainfall which made grass regrowth impossible. The herds died of starvation and, with them, the population dependent on their production. The introduction of what appeared to be a benign Western technology, one developed with humanitarian intent, interrupted a precarious ecological cycle and had severe human consequences.

This case illustration is offered, not as an argument for cessation of efforts to prolong or improve the lives of the handicapped, but in order to indicate that at each step we must be prepared for the secondary consequences of initial interventions. Better intensive care units for neonates clearly imply the demand for greater provision of medical, educational and social services for handicapped survivors and their families. There is little evidence that our society has recognized this consequence of the medical salvage operations which it is willing to support in acute care units.

Indeed, increasing biomedical sophistication — with its remarkable benefits in the management of acute illness — has diverted clinical attention from the chronic disorders which today constitute the major burden of morbidity in Western populations. The challenges, discouragements and the potential satisfactions for the physician are quite different in chronic care. Slowing an inevitably downhill course may be "all" that present methods permit. Bringing comfort to the patient and to the family in the face of death is a contribution of no mean proportion but one that is given insufficient attention in the training of physicians. Furthermore, measures to limit handicap and make life more tolerable do not change mortality statistics. Thus, it is a common criticism of contemporary medicine to say that it makes little difference because mortality tables have not changed over the past 20 years. The conclusion is false because mortality is not the relevant index in an era when chronic and degenerative disease has displaced acute life-threatening illness as the major public health challenge. Whether the doctor makes a difference can only be established by longitudinal studies of function in handicapped individuals treated in one or another way.

Questions of continuity and comprehensiveness of care bring us to the issues so cogently discussed in the paper by Dr. Pless. As he demonstrated, it is disappointingly difficult to obtain comprehensive and integrated services from the current medical system, whether the physician works in a team or as an individual practitioner. At stake are such questions as: what are the characteristics of students who enter medicine? How does the physician see his/her role? How is that role structured by society?

I know of no evidence that a better grounding in the humanities will yield more "humanistic" physicians than our present preference for science majors. Physicians should be educated men and women; a meaningful education must include the liberal arts. But does anyone seriously contend that, as a group, professors of English literature are more concerned with mankind than professors of physics? I am prepared to support the liberalization of premedical and medical education for itself but without any expectation that it will guarantee humane and sensitive physicians.

Quite a different perspective on the selection process is provided by the measures employed in the People's Republic of China. As it is described [4], nomination for medical school begins with fellow workers in the factory or the commune who select individuals on the basis of their service to the community. Whether the process in actuality corresponds to the theory, we do not know. But if we examine the concept and transpose it to the American scene, might we not consider requiring as a condition for entry into medical school several years of public service, say, in an inner city or rural health service, with the performance of the student evaluated in part by the consumers he/she served? That might be a requirement in addition to academic proficiency. Consumers don't want inept physicians. But we can anticipate that they would attend to compassion as well as intelligence. As faculties, we have not been very good at either selecting for or nurturing compassion. Consumer input might be of great assistance in the selection, if not the nuture.

The second point that Dr. Pless emphasized was the need for a reorganization of the methods of financing medical care. At present, there are financial disincentives for personal services. Consider the fee-for-service reimbursement under Medicare. Procedures (electrocardiograms, chest plates, diathermy treatment, etc.), which may take little physician time, are reimbursed without regard to the competence of the physician who employs them. Patient visits, whether they are brief or long, are paid at a standard rate. One need not suppose that physicians are venal, but merely human. If one loses income by listening for a half hour to the human concerns of the patient, it demands that the physician ignore self-interest in order to fulfill his clinical obligation. What is needed is a scheme that will reward the doctor for taking time when time is needed, and not penalize him. We need ways of paying surgeons for not operating as well as operating, ways of rewarding hospitals for not admitting patients who can be cared for on an ambulatory basis, and the like. The structure of the system must be altered to reinforce the behaviors society considers to be desirable. Restructuring the organization of medical care is likely to have a more decisive impact than attending only to medical training as a way of modifying physician behavior [5].

Beyond questions of student selection and the organization of medical practice, there is a more fundamental issue. The success of the biomedical enterprise in the past century has created a false paradigm of health care: the physician as an applied scientist who identifies and corrects the derangements in the patient's biologic machinery. The philosophical error is identified with the dichotomy between mind and body enunciated by Rene Descartes. That separation was pragmatic when it was introduced because it freed biology to study the body by reassuring the church that science would not tamper with the soul. But it has come to be a major barrier in the reintroduction of soul or mind into medicine.

To overstate the case, patients suffer "illnesses;" physicians diagnose and treat "diseases." I use illness to mean an experience of an uncomfortable change in state and/or an unwanted impairment in social performance. I use disease to mean an abnormality in the structure and/or function of body organs and systems, the definition employed by biomedicine.

So defined, illness and disease do not stand in a one-to-one relationship with one another. Disease may occur in the absence of illness. The person with hypertension may have no symptoms and therefore no illness. The physician who measures blood pressure expresses concern and prescribes medication. If the patient takes the medication, the side effects may make him ill. In his view, he entered the office well and left sick. He may stop the medicine, despite what he has been told about its value in reducing future risk. Only when the hypertension leads to heart failure or stroke does the person become a patient in his own eyes and agree with his doctor that he is sick. Even then, the agreement may be illusory in that both recognize a problem but differ in their view of it.

Organ pathology similar or even identical in degree may generate quite different reports of distress in different patients. In a study of outpatients with otitis media, Irish patients had fewer complaints than Italians although the findings on physical examination were similar [6]. Beecher, in a comparison of patients with similar traumatic injuries (one group battle casualties and the other automobile accident victims) [7], found that the soldiers required much less morphine than the civilian casualties.

Illness experience is patterned by culture. Medical lore is integral to every existing human culture. Every human group has a body of beliefs about illness and healing. As culture evolves over time, folk knowledge becomes the special prerogative of healers. The shaman or healer in traditional societies does what the physician does in Western societies. He diagnoses, he prescribes ritual actions designed to overcome illness; he casts a prognosis; and he legitimates the mysteries of death. He names and explains just as we name and explain, although he and we employ very different explanatory systems.

As medicine becomes professionalized (and this comment applies to learned practitioners of Eastern medical systems as well as to our own), the practitioner gets further and further removed from his client and less and less responsive to his client's perceptions of illness. In contrast, the indigenous healers were more sensitive to the personal and social aspects of illness because these were the aspects in which they could intervene — whereas we can affect the biology of illness. Our success in dealing with acute disease feeds the conceptual error that a technical fix is the potential solution to all illness problems. It would be absurd to suggest that we forego the power of biomedical methods. What requires emphasis is a parallel understanding of illness — chronic illness in particular — as psychosocial process. Our worship of restricted disease models resembles a ritual or magical belief more than it does scientific logic.

Models of illness, like models of physics, are ways of constructing reality, of imposing meaning on the chaos of the phenomenal world. There *is* a physical reality but it doesn't present itself to us organized in the ways we come to view it. The models we employ have decisive effects on our behavior. Those models determine the data we gather. Phenomena become *data* precisely because of their relevance to the sets of questions we choose to ask. Once in place, models act to generate their own verification by excluding from consideration phenomena that are outside of our frame of reference. Models are indispensable but they have an inherent toxicity because they can be mistaken for reality itself, rather than be seen as only one way of organizing that reality.

Error is compounded when abstractions are reified and diseases regarded as things. This was recognized by the founder of cellular pathology, Virchow, when he wrote [8]: "Diseases are not self-subsistent, circumscribed, autonomous organisms; they represent only the course of physiological phenomena under altered conditions." Even within the definition of disease as organ pathology, disease is not an entity but a relational concept. If disease is viewed as a relation, one can then choose those aspects of the relation most easily manipulated. Theory thus becomes an instrument of action [9]. One chooses a theory to highlight the variables most easily subject to influence.

There is much to be learned from the study of healing practices in other cultures in order to identify what it is that the patient seeks from the doctor. Healers have held an honored place in society for millenia although powerful surgical and medical technologies have been available for less than a century. This indicates that the ability to bring relief from suffering is inherent in the social structure of healing practices. Our contemporary preoccupation with the purely biologic aspects of clinical practice had led us to ignore the equally powerful psychosocial determinants of health and illness [10].

Symptom relief can be purchased at too heavy a price. The outcomes that matter are long range as well as episodic. The most effective medical encounter is one that not only brings relief but enhances the patient's ability to cope on his own.

The therapeutic benefit derived from medical presence, I contend, is evidence for the mediating role of psychosocial factors in the genesis and maintenance, as well as repair, of illness experience. In a given case, these factors may hold stage center or be peripheral to the main drama. They are never absent in the ill person until consciousness lapses; even then, they continue to operate in the responses of family and community. For most of its history, healing theory and practice have responded to psychosocial factors in symbolic and tacit ways; what is called for now is systematic social and behavioral research in medicine, supported by resources comparable in magnitude to those we have so profitably devoted to the biomedical enterprise. There can be no pretense that we yet possess methods of like investigative elegance and power. Equally, there need be no reason to doubt our ability to fashion such methods once we acknowledge how key they are to understanding contemporary health problems.

REFERENCES

1. Laurence, K. M.: Effect of early surgery for spina bifida cystica on survival and quality of life. Lancet 1:301–304, 1974.
2. McDermott, W.: Measuring the physician and his technology. Daedalus. (In press.)
3. Ormerod, W. E.: Ecological effect of control of African trypanosomiasis. Science 191:815–821, 1976.
4. Wen, C. P. and Hays, C. W.: Medical education in China in the postcultural revolution era. N. Eng. J. Med. 292:998–1005, 1975.
5. Friedson, E.: "Professional Dominance." New York: Atherton Press, 1970.
6. Zola, I. K.: Culture and symptoms: an analysis of patients' presenting complaints. Am. Sociol. Rev. 31:615–630, 1966.
7. Beecher, H. K.: Relationship of the significance of wound to the pain experienced. JAMA 161:1609–1613, 1956.
8. Virchow, R.: "Disease, Life and Man." Stanford: Stanford University Press, 1958.
9. Engelhardt, H. T.: Explanatory models in medicine: Facts, theories and values. Texas Rep. Biol. Med. 32:225–239, 1974.
10. Kleinman, A. M.: The cognitive structure of traditional medical systems. Ethnomedicine 3:27–45, 1974.